FITTER
FASTER

Your best ever body
in 8 weeks

DAVID KINGSBURY

SEVEN DIALS

CONTENTS

PART 3: MOVEMENT 182

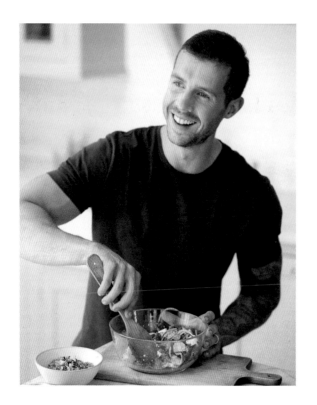

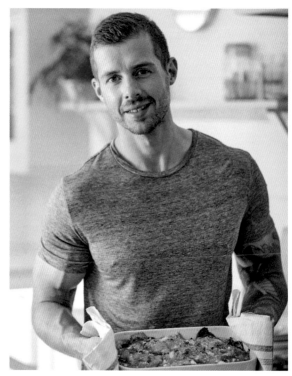

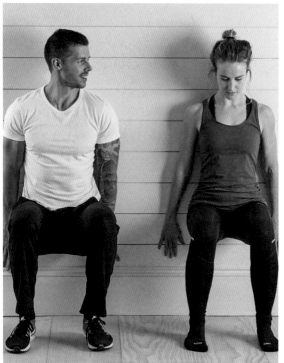

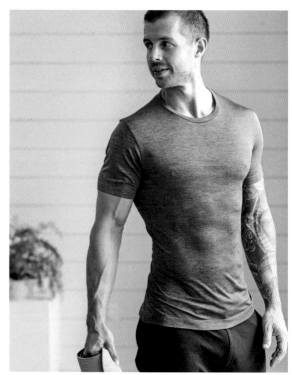

HELLO!

What is the difference between success and failure?

The answer is simple. It's having the correct formula to guarantee you results.

I'm David Kingsbury, a personal trainer in the film industry and beyond. Thank you for buying *Fitter Faster*, the only book that has been personalised for you to achieve the results you want. My work in the film industry doesn't accept anything but the best, and neither should you.

While some aspects of my career have been unusual – from red carpet premieres and working on film sets to leading sessions at trailer gyms in random car park locations – my passion for results remains the same as it was starting out in the industry over a decade ago. I know the demands of everyday life. I know how hard it can be to fit healthy eating and exercise into the chaos of each day. The focus for me is on providing a lifestyle solution, one that can easily fit around your daily commitments and still deliver sustainable results.

The film industry work is a big part of what I do, but my aim is to help as many people as possible. For me it isn't about big Hollywood budgets; it's about achieving amazing results no matter who you are.

I've put all my knowledge, all my experience and all my drive into this book. It's a journey you can choose to join me on, but if you make the commitment it's one you won't want to end. Let's do it together.

THE PREMISE

Your own personalised nutrition plan
+ your own personal fitness plan = success

I don't think I'm doing myself a disservice to say that *Fitter Faster* is a diet and exercise book like no other. I have packed in over a decade of personal training and nutritional knowledge within these pages to help create the best version of you.

Through all the incredible experiences I've had as a personal trainer and the thousands of people I've had the pleasure of working with, there has been a basic principle underlying everything I do. I strongly believe in a personalised approach. When it comes to health and fitness, I don't think there is a 'one-size-fits-all' plan that really works long-term. There can't be – because, as people, we come in different sizes, shapes, heights and body types. We all have different lifestyles and different goals and, wherever we are on our fitness journey, we're all starting from, and going to, a different place. Generic approaches aren't calculated to succeed, so let's not waste time looking for them.

Unlike most diet books, *Fitter Faster* takes those differences into consideration to treat you like an individual; looking at your body, your lifestyle and your goals to provide a bespoke solution that works. This isn't a random collection of low-calorie meals with some basic exercises; there are plenty of other books for you if that's all you want. This book is different because it's built on the solid foundation of custom nutrition that helps you not only hit your goals, but smash them out of the park: through delivering delicious recipes tailored to your goals. This means you can enjoy your food, happy in the knowledge that the calories and macros (see page 36 for an explanation of this) have been accurately calculated for you. With the recipes in this book, I've taken the guesswork out and put the flavour in . . . and they get results!

Paired with the achievable and focused training schedules, you no longer need to rely on luck to get in shape. I've got the formula for you and it works. Enjoy!

WHO AM I?

I'm YOUR personal trainer.

I've been a personal trainer to both celebrities and regular people like you and me for over a decade, but fitness has always been in my DNA: my father and grandfather developed fitness testing equipment for British Cycling in the 1980s, when the team started to dominate the sport worldwide. When I was 17, studying at college and deciding what to do next, a friend of mine told me he'd recently become a personal trainer, and that it might be a good match for me. It would allow me to work at something I loved, while still being able to get my own training in when I could. It sounded like the best of both worlds.

Before this conversation, I had never even heard of a 'personal trainer'. This was 2005 and personal training wasn't anywhere near as common as it is now. Successful trainers were few and far between, which made it a great time to be starting out. Initially I worked in gyms, then at a private PT studio. Not long after, I decided to go it alone and very fortunately I was able to get my hands on a space at Pinewood Studios in Buckinghamshire.

Given that my gym was at a film studio, it wasn't long before everyone and anyone from the cast and crew who worked on the film sets came by to exercise. Over time, my reputation began to grow. I trained one of the crew on *Snow White and the Huntsman* and they put my name forward to the powers that be. Soon I was training a couple of the stars of that movie.

I have always been so motivated that I rarely gave myself much time to reflect on where I was, or what I was doing, until the time I was working on the set of *Les Misérables*. At one point, we had almost the whole cast of the film in the gym. Big cast, small studio! It was a very surreal experience for me at the time. I remember taking a step back and looking around at all these actors in my gym and thinking to myself, 'Is this real?' That was the beginning of my journey with many famous actors that continues to date. I've worked on the set of some fantastic movies including *Assassin's Creed*, *Life*, *The Huntsman*, *Pan*, *Heart of the Sea*, *X-Men* and *The Wolverine* to name just a few.

The work I do with actors might sound glamorous, and it has its perks, but the real work is done in the gym and the kitchen: early mornings, late nights, long days, hard work, the right food and complementary training plans. Today, my experience on film sets means I often get called the 'Hollywood trainer'. It sounds great, but the truth is I do more work in Buckinghamshire car parks than I do in Tinsel Town!

None of the people I work with would come back if I didn't know my stuff or failed to deliver on what I say I can. People often think celebrities have it easy with their chefs, stylists and Hollywood budgets, but the truth is they have the same problems as the rest of us. We all have challenges we have to overcome if we want to succeed. Support can be one of the most important parts of any plan. Even if someone has the best training and diet programme in the world, if they are unable to follow it, it will be ineffective. My job as a trainer is to be there for my clients in the form of motivation, encouragement and simply understanding and accepting their individual challenges. You will find a lot of encouragement in the pages of this book as well as from the inspiring and supportive #TeamKingsbury online community.

I may be best known for my film work, which isn't surprising seeing as the bodies I have transformed have been on the big screen for millions of people to see. For me, though, it's all those people you've never heard of who are following my plans and getting extraordinary results that make my job so satisfying. Maybe my next proudest achievement will be to work with you and help you achieve your personal best.

HOW TO USE THIS BOOK

I have put everything I know into this book to help make you everything you want to be.

In *Fitter Faster*, I have simplified my techniques to make them easy to use, but without losing their effectiveness. If you find words or phrases you don't understand, don't worry: everything I talk about is defined in the Key Words and Terms section (page 261) at the back of the book. Trust me, it'll be second nature in no time.

Before we get started, let's just clarify how it's all going to work:

- ☐ Read up about how the plan works in **Part 1: Your plan** (page 12).
- ☐ Fill in your goals and what you want to achieve from the next eight weeks (page 23).
- ☐ Calculate and find out your daily calorie budget and which recipe menu to follow in **Part 2: Food** (page 34).
- ☐ Read about the training plans available and decide on the one you are going to follow in **Part 3: Movement** (page 182).
- ☐ Armed with your goals, menus and training plans, you can begin!

Are you ready to get fitter, faster?
Perfect. Let's do this!

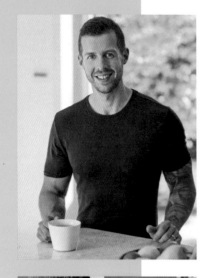

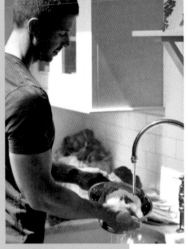

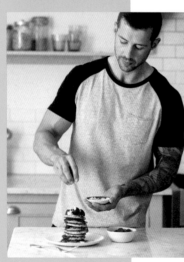

PART 1:

YOUR PLAN

WHY DIETS FAIL BUT YOU WILL SUCCEED

How many diets have you tried in your life?

How many diets do you think your friends have tried? Your family? Work colleagues? Neighbours? Don't be embarrassed. The number is pretty high for all of us! Now ask yourself this: how many of them have had a lasting impression on your weight? Those diets might have worked in the short term, but health and fitness is a long-term undertaking.

Most of us have been victims of the latest fad diet at some point in our lives. One that promised incredible weight loss through only eating soup, or cheeseburgers, or sand or whatever crazy notion was at its core. We follow them because we want to look our best on holiday in our budgie-smugglers or bikini. We want to get into that dress for a friend's wedding or slim down just to keep up with our kids. Well, there's a way to do it successfully and it doesn't involve crazy diets or unsubstantiated, miraculous claims from flashy, faceless websites.

To make a positive change to your lifestyle and to drop body fat takes discipline – and knowledge. So let's start by looking at why, as a population, we are gaining body fat.

#1: WE'RE EATING MORE JUNK FOOD

Who doesn't like a takeaway every now and again? I know I certainly do. There's nothing wrong with some junk food occasionally, but for many of us, 'occasionally' happens all too often. We all have hectic lives: work commitments, family dramas, taxi-driving for the kids, our own stressful commute and our online lives all take their toll. By the time we settle down after a busy day, the last thing we want to do is cook. But the recipes in this book will make it easy!

#2: OUR SUGAR CONSUMPTION IS SOARING A lot

of the extra calories we're eating come from processed foods. Sugar, in all its many forms and disguises, plays a large part in processed foods, which means we're eating it even when we might not realise we're doing so.

Sugar is a key factor when it comes to obesity. In our bodies, the part of us which is in charge of regulating our energy balance is the brain. It's the brain that ensures we know when to eat so we don't starve and also the organ that tries to stop us accumulating excess fat. Our brains don't 'register' sugary, fatty, heavily processed foods in the same way as other foods, we don't get the same *I'm full* signals. This means that we tend to eat more than we normally would.

There's a phrase that you should look out for and avoid like a saccharine plague. It's 'added sugar'. Eating excessive amounts of added sugar can have harmful effects on your metabolism, which can lead to insulin resistance, belly fat, fatty liver disease and heart disease.Likewise, the brain doesn't 'register' sugar in its liquid form in the same way it registers solid sugar. If you drink a lot of sugary drinks, your brain doesn't automatically make you eat fewer calories to compensate. It's the reason why liquid sugar calories are usually added *on top* of the daily calorie intake. Many people are aware of the high sugar content in carbonated drinks, but often fruit juices are no better, despite their healthy-looking packaging.

#3: WE GAIN WEIGHT EACH YEAR . . . WHICH WE MAY NEVER GET RID OF People who are overweight don't become

that way overnight. Weight gain happens slowly over weeks, months, years. As well as this gradual increase, at certain points in our lives – think new job, kids, stressful/ emotional times – we may gain more weight and not always realise it. Likewise, holidays such as Christmas, Easter and our well-deserved summer holidays are when we tend to binge on all those 'treat' foods, chocolates, alcohol and sugary soft drinks.

In many ways it seems perfectly natural that we overdo it a little at those times. The problem is that some of us may not ever lose the weight we gain then: if I gain 2 kg over Christmas, but only lose 1 kg when I go back to 'normal' and then repeat that pattern over time, you can see where the problem lies. But with a little guidance, we can all rustle up good food in less time than you might think.

#4: WE HAVE AN OFFICE CULTURE Many people blame
the rise in obesity levels on the decrease of physical activity. It's true that most
of us should be exercising more often, but I don't think it's as simple as that. As a
population we tend to have jobs that aren't physically demanding – and most of
us are stuck behind a computer all day. So even if you do manage to go to the gym
three times a week, you may hardly be moving the other four days. Our bodies are
simply not meant for these levels of inactivity.

Our energy balance is the number one factor when it comes to changing our
body shape. The primary reason we are gaining body fat is the simple truth that
we are consuming more calories than we are burning off in exercise. Later in the
book I will show you how to understand your own personal energy demands so
you can ensure you get this important factor right for *your* body. For now, just
remember that '*calories are king*'.

So, bearing all this in mind, why do the fad diets of the world fail?

- **They're not sustainable. Faddy diets try to counteract the effects of**
junk food, excess calories and lack of activity. But most diets are simply not
designed to be sustainable; instead they are created to 'shock' the body into
losing weight in a relatively short period of time. Even if they do work in the
short term, if they suck the fun out of meal times, they are less likely to become
the cornerstone of your personal nutrition. You need a plan that is sustainable:
think less 'crash dieting', more 'healthy living'.
- **They're not tailored to your needs. There is no one-size-fits-all**
approach to food, although a lot of people promote this! In order for a diet to
work it has to know you and understand your body and goals, and it also has to
adapt as your body changes. A fundamental flaw with most food plans is that
they stay the same week in, week out. What we need today to lose body fat may
not be the same as what we need in four weeks' time, working at the same rate.
As our weight drops, so does our calorie requirement.
- **Healthy recipes can be deceiving when it comes to calorie content.**
You can still overeat healthy foods or drinks and gain weight, even if they
are full of 'good' ingredients. Healthy foods are not calorie-exempt. A lot of

health-food cookery books or recipes supply snacks and meals with 'healthy ingredients', yet they are incredibly calorie-dense. That makes it very easy to overdo your daily calories.

- **Harsh diets can have a negative effect on your long-term fat loss.**
Yo-yo and crash diets that are designed to shock your body into weight loss can have a negative impact on your long-term fat loss. Weight lost will invariably creep back on after a crash diet, and often people will end up exceeding the weight they started at.Furthermore, the cycle of losing weight and gaining weight can be accompanied by biological changes that you won't necessarily be aware of. If you drop your calories too low or lose and gain weight often, you may have undergone some adaptive metabolic changes. They can potentially mean that you will expend slightly less energy than you would expect based on standard calorie calculations – in other words, you may have to work even harder to lose weight in future!

Lifestyle will always win

So fad or crash diets don't work in the long term. But there is one other important thing to remember: you can't 'out-train' a bad diet either. Some people think that they can eat what they want as long as they go to the gym a few times a week. Sadly, that's not the case. The truth is that to achieve your goals you have to eat in a way that supports and nurtures them specifically, whatever they are. If your goals change, so too will the food you need to eat to continually achieve them.

The focus of this book is not to get you to drop weight over eight weeks just for the sake of it; instead it's a way you can eat and exercise the right way forever! Sure, you'll see the results in a short time, but the idea is that you'll learn some things that will stand you in good stead for the rest of your life.

THE SCIENCE OF RESULTS

The more you read about a topic, particularly online, the more confusing it can become.

With the amount of misinformation available on the web and in the media, even the simplest of topics can be shrouded in contradiction and vagaries. Health and fitness is no different, but I want to change that.

I'm sure we all know that you need a certain amount of energy (in the form of calories) just to stay alive. You can get this energy from the food you eat, or you can retrieve it from stored energy (e.g. your fat tissue). To change your weight you need an imbalance between energy intake and energy expenditure.

In theory, it looks like this:

- If you eat fewer calories than you expend, you will lose weight.
- If you do the opposite (i.e. eat more calories than you burn off), you will gain weight.
- If you expend the same as you eat, you'll maintain weight.

Sounds pretty simple right? Well, in theory 'yes' but there is also the influence of weight, age and height plus more changeable variables, like sex hormone levels, exercise style, medication use, genetic predisposition and gut bacteria, not to mention many more individual factors that are harder to accurately calculate and often unique to each person. Nevertheless the best place to start when calculating your calorific needs is your activity level.

To give you an idea of how exercise levels affect your body's needs a friend of mine, Gary, and I recently compared our calorie needs for this plan. On face value, we're quite similar: we're both men, he weighs 87 kg, and I weigh 85 kg. But because Gary exercises one to two hours a week and I exercise five plus, his daily calorie requirement for fat loss is 1,659 per day, whereas mine is 2,496. If I were put on a plan with his needs, i.e. 1,659 calories per day, I would suffer. I'd potentially lose muscle, not be able to function well and I'd also be hungry too often. This would negatively impact my ability to stick to the plan and I would no doubt fall off the wagon and raid my daughter's snack cupboard, slowing down my progress. Similarly, if you put Gary on my plan, i.e. 2,496 calories per day, he would not lose fat effectively.

Individualised calorie intake is the most important factor here, but calories aren't the only factor that need to be considered. Our macronutrients – what make up the calorie content of our food – should also be tailored to our needs. Macronutrients come in three categories: carbohydrates, protein and fat. With only one to two hours of exercise per week, Gary's body's demand for carbohydrates is less than mine. In addition, his body may not be as toleratant of carbohydrates. I generally determine this from body fat percentage or waist/height ratio (in this book we will use a waist measurement to determine yours; see page 37). Because he is less active and carries more body fat around his midsection, he requires fewer carbs and has less ability to process and use them effectively. So we both also have a different need for carbohydrates.

So, while we all share the basic equation for energy in and out, the factors that make it work are going to be different for each and every one of us. This book will provide a personalised approach to get the balance right for you. When we want to lose weight we can influence our energy demands on both sides of the equation to give us the results we want.

ENERGY IN

Food contains energy, but we absorb fewer calories from minimally processed foods than we do from highly processed foods, because the latter are easier to digest. In simple terms, the more 'processed' a food is, the more digestion work has already been done for you, and let's not forget that highly processed foods are generally less filling, more energy-dense and are consequently more likely to cause overeating. Make a meal from scratch and your body has to work harder to digest it. What this also means is the calories on food labels aren't necessarily accurate compared with the figures a nutritionist would give you.

ENERGY OUT

'Energy out' refers to the energy burned through moving around. We might eat the same foods, but we all expend energy differently and to varying degrees. A large part of energy out is burned by our Resting Metabolic Rate (RMR), which is the number of calories you burn each day while at rest. This includes the calories you expend just breathing in and out, thinking about your next big idea and generally staying alive. How much depends on other factors such as your weight, body composition, gender and age, to name a few. For example, if you are carrying 20 kg more body weight than someone else who is the same age, height and gender, with identical activity levels, then it's likely your daily calorie expenditure will be considerably higher.

In addition to the RMR, Non-Exercise Activity Thermogenesis (NEAT) is concerned with the calories you burn through fidgeting, standing and staying upright and all other physical activities (with the exception of purposeful exercise). NEAT, too, varies from person to person and also changes from day to day.

Lastly – and potentially most importantly – we have physical activity. Physical activity burns calories, and the amount and intensity of that physical activity will greatly affect your calorie expenditure.

MAKING YOUR PLAN

Right, I've promised you a plan that's tailored to you, so let's do it! By following this three-step process you'll be in the best possible place to get fitter, faster.

STEP 1: SET YOUR GOALS

Without a set goal, we have neither a way of devising a plan to achieve it, nor the understanding of why we are doing it. So throughout this journey, you're going to be setting yourself some short-, medium- and long-term goals. Whatever those goals are, they will be very personal and unique to you. We all have different issues to address so we all have different targets to hit.

In order to improve body composition, fat loss is the quickest route to change. Fat loss from person to person will vary. If someone is very overweight they have more fat to lose and can safely and easily lose more than someone who has less to lose. We won't be assessing fat loss through measuring fat mass on this plan due to the challenges of getting accurate measurements. Instead, we'll be measuring weight loss – it's much easier and also more reliable.

Have a think about what you'd like your goals to be – and make sure they're realistic. Here are some guidelines for the weight-loss goals you could set yourself:

- For weight loss, 2 lbs/1 kg a week is often considered the healthy standard – a middle ground for results. If you are only marginally overweight or just looking to trim up a bit, then aiming for less than 2 lbs/1 kg would be more suitable. You could think of aiming for 1 lb/0.5 kg per week.
- If, however, you are very overweight then aiming for more than 2 lbs/1 kg per week is a very realistic goal. Depending on your starting weight you could potentially aim for a loss of 2–4 lbs/1–2 kg each week.
- Clothing sizes and measurements can be a useful tool for tracking progress so feel free to make these your focus if you prefer .

You will see overleaf a page called 'My Motivator Page' where you can write your goals down so you can remember them. Often people say results don't happen overnight, but in some ways they do. Each small step you take every day will bring a small amount of progress, and this progress adds up to smashing your big goal! But also remember that if you are unable to follow the plan for a day, it doesn't matter – leave it behind and focus on getting the next day right.

THE SCALES

Weighing yourself, especially at the beginning of a diet plan, can be tough and a little demotivating if you don't see what you want to see. We often hate what the scales tell us, but let's start to think of it differently. Weighing ourselves on this plan is about setting a metric and allowing us to calculate our calories. It is a tool for progress and an important one at that. It is a measure of progress to an extent but it is more a measure to *ensure* progress. So instead of dreading stepping on the scales, start seeing them as your best friend – they are going to get you where you want to go!

STEP 2: CALCULATE YOUR CALORIE BUDGET

I've said it before, but calories are the number one deciding factor when it comes to achieving your results. If you skipped the section on 'The Science of Results' (page 17), then I'd recommend you go back and take a look. The number of calories you consume each day needs to be specific to your body type and goals, so this is the most important part of this book. To do this you need to first decide how much activity you're going to do.

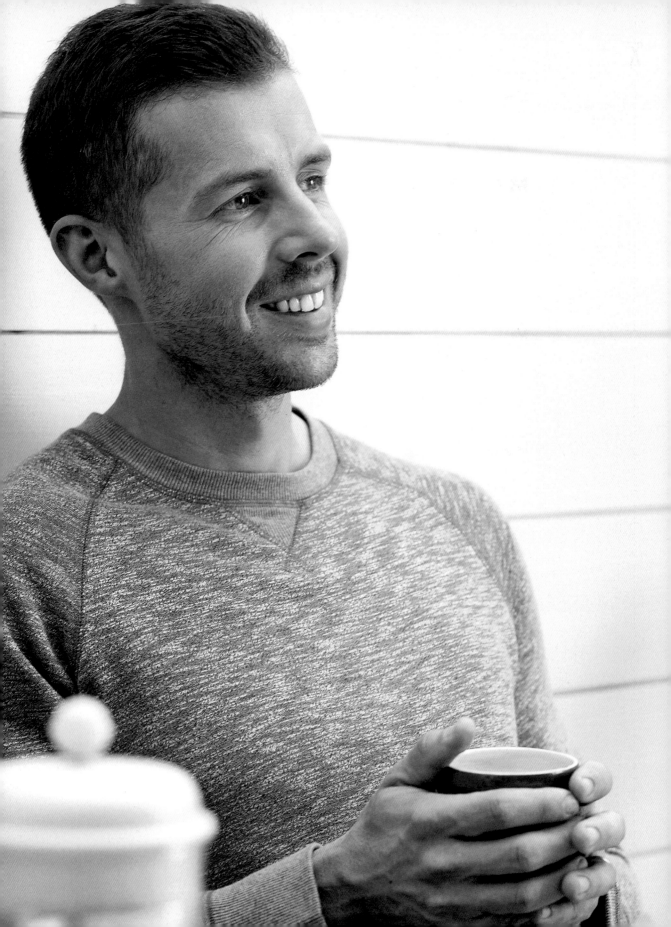

As you read through parts 1 and 2 you'll find prompts to write your goals down here – as well as how you're going to reach them – and some space to track your progress. I'd recommend cutting it out and pinning it somewhere you'll see it every day, such as on the fridge.

MY MOTIVATOR PAGE

I currently weigh _____ kg and am a clothes size _____.

In eight weeks from now, _____ [insert date], I want to have lost at least _____ kg of weight and to drop to a size _____.

My activity level is _____ and I plan to do _____ hours of exercise per week.

I will keep track of my weight, measurements and menus here:

	Beginning	Week 2	Week 4	Week 6	Week 8
Weight in kg					
Waist measurement					
Menu colour:					
Breakfast					
Lunch					
Dinner					
Snack code					
Carb snack? (Y/N)					

To be successful, I need to:
- Get eight hours' sleep a night
- Eat from the food plan
- Stick to my movement plan

WHAT'S YOUR ACTIVITY LEVEL?

Take a look at the options below and decide which level you want to commit to for the following eight weeks. Exercise here covers any and all hard physical activity. Include hours of gym sessions, home workouts, cardio sessions, fitness classes, swimming, cycling to work, etc. You can achieve results with limited activity time but adding exercise will help ensure positive body composition changes and improved health. Adding movement also allows you to eat a higher number calories each week and still make progress.

Level 1: 1–3 hours of exercise per week
Level 2: 3–5 hours of exercise per week
Level 3: 5+ hours of exercise per week

Now add this to the Motivator Page (page 23).

A note on the activity levels above: we all lead different lifestyles, and some of us burn more calories day to day than others, even without additional deliberate exercise. If you work a 9–5 office job, and go for the occasional short walk in the evenings and the weekends, the activity levels above will work for you. However, if you have a physical job that keeps you on your feet, or when you get home from work you never sit still and go for long hikes at the weekend, you will be burning more calories. If this is you, bump yourself up a level. For example, if you only do 1 hour of deliberate exercise a week but work as a gardener, use Activity Level 2. Or if you do 3 hours exercise a week and go for day-long walks every weekend, use Activity Level 3.

YOUR FAT-LOSS FORMULA

Taking your current weight and the activity level you've just decided upon, use the appropriate formula from the choices overleaf and round your calories to the nearest 100. The resulting figure will give you the number of calories you need to eat each day to lose fat. (Don't worry about the rounding; eating 50 calories over your calculated figure will not prevent you from losing weight.)

FAT-LOSS CALORIES, MALE

Level 1 (hours of exercise per week: 1–3)
Your weight in kg × 12.0 + 615 = Fat-loss calories

Level 2 (hours of exercise per week: 3–5)
Your weight in kg × 14.8 + 765 = Fat-loss calories

Level 3 (hours of exercise per week: 5+)
Your weight in kg × 18.3 + 940 = Fat-loss calories

FAT-LOSS CALORIES, FEMALE

Level 1 (hours of exercise per week: 1–3)
Your weight in kg × 8.1 + 650 = Fat-loss calories

Level 2 (hours of exercise per week: 3–5)
Your weight in kg × 10.5 + 840 = Fat-loss calories

Level 3 (hours of exercise per week: 5+)
Your weight in kg × 12.9 + 1035 = Fat-loss calories

Let's look at an example. If I were doing it for myself then, as an 85 kg man who exercises more than 5 hours per week, I would use the Level 3 formula for men:

85 × 18.3 + 940 = 2496 calories per day (let's round that up to 2500)

If I reduced my activity levels to 3–5 hours of exercise each week then the calculation would use the Level 2 formula:

85 × 14.8 + 765 = 2023 calories per day (let's round that down to 2000)

As you can see here, the level of activity you can commit to is very important in selecting your calories, so pick a level you believe you can maintain. Now it's your turn . . .

_____ × _____ = _____

(Weight in kg)   (Choose from formulas above)   (calories)

Now round your calories up or down to the nearest 100. This is your starting calorie budget. Add this to the Motivator Page (page 23)

N.B. If your calorie calculation gives you a number that is below 1200 calories then it suggests you are quite light and have low levels of activity. If that is the case, 1200 calories a day will likely still be a calorie deficit for you, albeit a smaller one. This is actually preferable for you as a lighter individual and you may not be looking to drop as much weight each week. If you would like to increase your calorie deficit, then you can also increase your activity level to do so.

Remember, don't go BELOW your calorie recommendation; not only is this unhealthy, but you'll probably only get hungry and cheat!

WHY THE FORMULAS WORK

As part of my online fitness and nutrition plans, I have researched methods of calculating calorific needs based on individual characteristics of a person (age, weight, height, gender), their level of exercise and their goals. I also have the experience of over ten years as a trainer with thousands of real life case studies. So what you might think are some quite random numbers in the formulas are actually the result of some very informed algorithms. I have refined this calculation over time and they deliver accurate figures for the people I train time and time again.

The three most crucial factors are weight, amount of exercise and gender. Other factors have an effect, but a minor one compared to these three. The formulas used in this book are a simplified version of a more refined model, but still produce answers accurate enough to give you a calorie budget to work from that will achieve your goals.

STEP 3: MAKING PROGRESS AND UPDATES

I'm not solely interested in your progress over the first week; I want you to make consistent progress week after week. At the core of any successful plan should be the ability for it to change with you and remain flexible. The calories and macros you need to drop body fat today will not necessarily be the same a month from now. And you don't want a plan that only works this month, but for months, even years, afterwards.

As we lose weight, our demand for calories decreases and as our body adjusts to our new diet and rebalances hormones, fat loss can slow down or even stop. At the same time, though, as we get leaner and fitter, our tolerance for carbohydrates increases. We also tend to become more insulin-sensitive, causing our body to produce less insulin, which can result in LESS fat storage and allowing more fatty acids to be burned off. Our bodies are complicated!

For these reasons, we'll be recalculating our calories every two weeks: it's going to be crucial in guaranteeing continued progress on your plan. To recalculate your calories, go back to the fat-loss formulas on page 26 and redo the calculation with your new weight. Then check whether you need a new menu colour (page 35). You should also measure your waist (page 37) to check whether you can add carb-based snacks to your plan. You can record all these numbers in the useful table on your Motivator Page (page 23), though of course you may want to extend your plan beyond eight weeks when you see how much progress you've made!

When you weigh yourself, do so at the same time you did for your first weigh-in at the beginning of the plan, and take the average over a few days, as your weight will naturally fluctuate by as much as one to two kg from day to day.

FINALLY . . .

BELIEVE IN YOURSELF! One of the biggest barriers to success
I have seen over the years is lack of personal commitment. If you are unsure of
whether something will work or not, that doubt, however small, makes it a lot
harder to go all in and fully commit to any challenge. Any doubt means you can
easily talk yourself out of the plan and back into your normal habits. This book
provides all the tools you need for effective fat loss. You can trust that it will work
for you. Stay committed and focused and you'll see the results for yourself. It won't
always be easy, but it will always be worth it!

BE CONSISTENTLY CONSISTENT Results come from
consistency, not all-out effort. They are achieved not through extreme changes, but
through steady, consistent work. Make this easy for yourself by not going too low on
your calories. If you cut them too much, or too quickly, you will open yourself up to
extreme hunger. It is almost impossible to follow a food plan if you are hungry all day
long. We all know what'll happen next. In addition, enjoy what you are eating! Luckily,
all the meals in this book are tried and tested and taste delicious.

TRAIN SMARTER Often, when people want to lose weight, their
immediate reaction is to increase their cardiovascular exercise. Successful fat-
loss training doesn't call for hours of exercise in the gym or marathon sessions
pounding the pavement. You simply have to balance your calories with your
activity. In fact in many cases, over-exercising can be a detriment to your fat-loss
efforts, due to the fact it can increase your cortisol levels and your appetite. The
training within the plan you're about to start is demanding, but it's also absolutely
achievable. It is the perfect balance of resistance and intensity, which will deliver
amazing body composition changes you'll be able to see.

RESULTS = MOTIVATION The single most motivating factor is
seeing your results right there in the mirror or in the photographs that you're in.

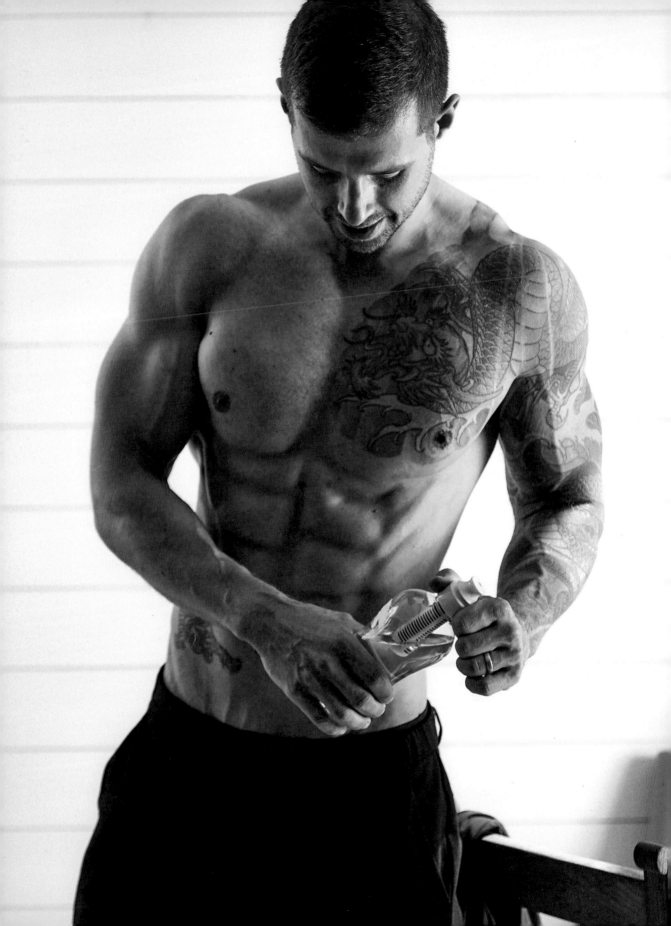

If you can keep motivation high and consistent then you have the formula for success right in front of you. On this plan you will see those results for yourself, which will drive you forwards and keep you motivated. You'll be making progress week after week and I can't wait see it. How? I'm glad you asked.

SHARING IS CARING
Support can sometimes be the fine line between success and failure. Having a team of people who will help motivate, inspire and support you through each and every step is something very special. I can give you that, or rather #TeamKingsbury can. Thousands of people make up this community, so come and see what is possible through their results and get support for your own journey. We'll only get stronger with you on board!

Instagram @TeamKingsbury #TeamKingsbury

Twitter @davidkingsbury #teamkingsbury

Goals set, mantras done – here we go!

CASE STUDY: **CAROLYN**

You are going to succeed with this plan, like the many people who have done so before you. So throughout this book, to keep you motivated, I want to show you just how effective my systems have been. First up, here's Carolyn, 27.

Weight lost: 19.8lbs/9kg
Exercise per week: 5-6 hours
Calories per day: 1500-1800
Reason for starting: I wanted a healthier lifestyle that was sustainable.

Have you tried losing weight before?
Plenty of times. Initially I would lose a little bit of weight, but I always found that after a little bit of time I would be right where I started as I couldn't maintain either the diet or exercise program long term for whatever reason.

How did you feel when you started the plan?
I was tired and just in a lousy mood most of the time. My weight had creeped up from bad habits and I felt that I had let stress take over parts of my life. I didn't feel like going anywhere besides home after work.

How do you feel now?
I have much more energy and feel healthier overall. My weight isn't something I think about as much anymore and I feel more focused on gaining strength and pushing myself harder.

What did you like the most in terms of following the plan?
The recipes were a big plus! Lots of choice and all really tasty.

What exercises did you like the most or find gave you the most results?

Weight training I think overall shaped up parts of my body and defined my stomach. My favourite thing was rowing sprints.

Was there anything you found tricky?

Eating a specific diet can be difficult, especially when treats are always around you at the office! I was firm that I wanted to complete the plan following both the diet and exercises though, so I stuck to my guns and passed on all those treats.

Will you keep going with the plan now?

Yes, definitely! I plan on working on gaining some muscle and strength for a while and then I will lean down for next spring for a holiday with my sister.

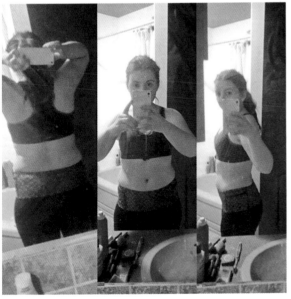

Week 1

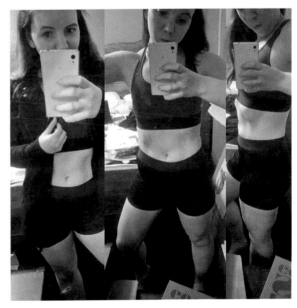

Week 8

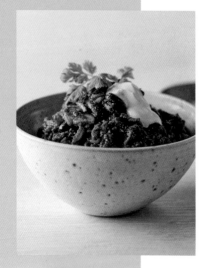

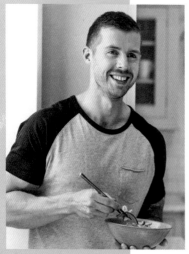

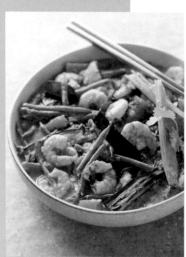

PART 2:
FOOD

SELECTING YOUR MENU

Now we're going to get into one of the most enjoyable parts of this plan: choosing your food! Before you start picking the recipes based on what you fancy, it's vital you understand how to select the menu that's going to work for you and your goals.

HOW THE MENUS WORK

Each recipe in this book comes in six portion sizes, each of which has its own colour. Your colour menu will depend on the calorie budget you calculated back on page 27.

Cals	Breakfast	Lunch	Dinner	Snack
≤ 1200	1	1	1	A
1300	2	1	1	A
1400	2	2	1	A
1500	2	2	2	A
1600	3	2	2	A
1700	3	3	2	A
1800	3	3	2	B
1900	3	3	3	B
2000	4	3	3	B

Cals	Breakfast	Lunch	Dinner	Snack
2100	4	4	3	B
2200	4	4	4	B
2300	5	4	4	B
2400	5	5	4	B
2500	5	4	4	2 x A
2600	5	5	4	2 x A
2700	5	5	5	2 x A
2800	6	5	5	2 x A
2900	6	6	5	2 x A
3000	6	6	6	2 x A

The rest is very simple: eat three meals per day. All the meals are interchangeable, so if you'd rather have three breakfasts or three dinners, you can – so long as they correspond to your colour menu, you'll see the same results. Equally, if you don't want to have three meals the same size, you can go down a level in one meal so that you can go up a level in another – the calories will still be the same.

Each snack has two portion sizes, A or B and how many you have will depend on your calorie allowance. See opposite for information on whether you can choose from the high-carb or the low-carb snack recipe selection.

So, as an example, if your calories are calculated at 1700, select any breakfast and lunch with yellow portion size, any dinner with orange portion size and any snack with the A portion size. Based on the selection above, you now have a personalised food plan that has been calculated to your needs! This approach to your nutrition will put you in an incredibly strong position for achieving results. Make a note of the colour menus you'll be starting with on the Motivator Page (page 23).

MACROS

Each meal contains the key three macronutrients: carbohydrates, protein and fat. These macros are split in a way that is most suited for fat loss for the vast majority of people, and all the recipes are built on advanced nutrition software so the margin for error is small.

The macros of your meals are as follows:

20 per cent of calories from carbohydrates

40 per cent of calories from proteins

40 per cent of calories from fats

This format focuses on a reduced carbohydrate level and favours fats and proteins for energy, which encourages fat loss. Keeping your carbs and insulin under control in my experience facilitates better fat loss.

For the best results, 'improved body composition' is what we are looking for. To achieve this we need to drop body fat and maintain muscle. This is where the protein comes in. Protein is very important for muscle maintenance during a fat-loss plan and keeping the levels high will ensure you keep hold of all that hard-earned muscle whilst you are losing body fat.

Your body needs energy to function and the fats provide the extra energy you need. Fat is often given a bad rep – 'fat makes you fat' – but this is simply not the truth. It gets this reputation as it contains the largest number of calories per gram of the three macros. But you will only get fat eating fat if your overall calories are too high. Fat is actually one of the secret weapons for effective fat loss, because it provides energy with the lowest impact on your blood sugar and insulin levels. On a biochemical level, eating the right fats makes your body more efficient at burning it.

CARB SNACKS OR NO CARB SNACKS

We all have different needs and tolerances to carbohydrates, so if your waist is over a certain measurement you will only be having the lower-carb snacks alongside your meals. If your waist is below the cut-off you will have high-carb snacks on the days when you do resistance work using weights (i.e. circuits, bodyweight training, weight training) and low-carb snacks every other day. N.B. only exercise in which you are using weights counts here – if you do other forms of exercise, such as cardiovascular or toning work, you should choose from the low-carb snacks on those days.

The reason for this cut-off is that if you have a certain amount of abdominal fat it is likely you are somewhat insulin insensitive. Consuming high-carb snacks therefore results in your body producing a large amount of insulin, a hormone which encourages fat storage and inhibits the breakdown of fatty acids. As you lose body fat, insulin sensitivity tends to increase, reducing the amount of insulin your body produces when consuming carbohydrates. Therefore, as body fat reduces, high-carb snacks can be introduced into the plan on days when you need the extra boost of ready energy, without the risk of a high increase in fat storage.

Waist measurement has been shown by medical research to be an excellent tool for predicting insulin resistance, regardless of height. While it is true that taller people in general have larger waists, the effect is small and complex. However, if you are very tall (over 6'4"/193cm), add an inch to the cut-off; if you are quite short (under 4'11"/150cm), subtract an inch.

HOW TO FIND YOUR WAIST MEASUREMENT

The cut-off for high-carb snacks are these waist measurements:
Male: 37 inches (94cm)
Female: 33 inches (84cm)

- Remove or raise any clothing to just below your chest.
- Use your fingers to find the top of your hips and the base of your ribcage.
- Find the midpoint between the two: this is your waist.
- Wrap the tape around your waist.
- Take your measurement while standing up straight and exhaling slowly.
- Repeat it, just to double-check your measurement. You can record it on the Motivator Page (page 23)

FAQS

Almost time for the recipes! But before I share them with you, here are some handy FAQs that will hopefully answer any questions you have about the food plans.

Q: HOW MANY MEALS SHOULD I BE HAVING A DAY AND WHEN SHOULD I BE EATING THEM?

A: A lot of people say it's important to eat a certain number of meals each day. The truth is, while certain people with very specific training goals may need to worry about food timing and frequency, for most of us the key aspect is hitting our daily calorie requirements and macro targets. Myths like 'eating late at night will make you fat' or 'eating more meals will affect your metabolism' are just not supported by evidence (as is the idea that you need to eat a constant supply of protein to keep building muscle).

Our bodies are in a state of constant flux, going from an anabolic state (i.e. building and repairing tissue during rest periods) to a catabolic state (breaking it down again). Because of that, it doesn't really matter when you eat or how often, it's the net balance over time that's important – in other words, whether you're in a calorie surplus or calorie deficit over a sustained period. A deficit will mean you lose weight; a surplus will mean you gain weight. It's that simple.

Intermittent fasting, however, can have very positive results. It's essentially an eating pattern that involves you cycling between a window of eating and one of fasting every day. It's not about a repetition of starving yourself and binge-eating, it's much more controlled than that. It isn't an integral part of the plan but if it's something you want to incorporate then see the box opposite.

INTERMITTENT FASTING

What is it?

Intermittent fasting focuses on improving your body's fat-burning potential and your hormonal response to food. While it might be an alien concept for humans to deliberately go without food for a little while, there are some real benefits to trying it, particularly on this plan, as it's a way of eating that will help accelerate your fat-loss results. Intermittent fasting tends to work better for men, but does have results for women too.

How does it work?

When you go for an extended period of time without eating, your body initiates a number of cellular repair processes – for example, it will remove waste materials from your cells. It will also alter your hormone levels, so your stored body fat is more accessible, which is where things get interesting. During the fasting stage, insulin levels in your bloodstream will significantly drop, which will help when it comes to fat burning. Whilst they drop, your human growth hormone will increase. This higher level will not only facilitate fat burning, but muscle gain too. Many of the potential benefits of intermittent fasting are built on these hormonal changes.

How do I do it?

Pick an eight-hour window if you're a man and a 10–12-hour one if you're a woman, which remains consistent every day. Eat all your food and snacks within this window and don't consume any calories outside of this window. Do your best to stick within it when you can; this will ensure you get the most benefits, but if you have to break this rule every now and then, it's not a big deal.

There are certain situations in which I'd suggest you avoid intermittent fasting altogether:

- If you have high cortisol levels
- If you suffer from high levels of stress
- If you cannot fit your eating window into your family routine
- If you suffer from or have suffered from eating disorders
- If you normally eat breakfast very early
- If you train for long-duration sessions in your fasting period
- If you are a woman and experience problems with your menstrual cycles

Intermittent fasting can help deliver fat-loss results but it won't work for everyone. What will work is calculated and controlled calories, so don't worry if you don't get on with it. It isn't going to make or break your results.

Q: WHAT SORT OF MEALS WILL I BE EATING? I CAN'T DO YET ANOTHER RABBIT-FOOD PLAN!

A: I wholeheartedly believe food doesn't have to be boring to be nutritious. People stick to boring 'healthy' recipes because they know they can trust that they are working. But you can only tolerate them for so long before you get so bored you cave in and order a takeaway. The great thing about this plan is that not only can you trust them but you can also try all the recipes in the book, whatever colour category you're in, so you have a huge choice to suit all tastes. In addition, all recipes are high in protein and avoid fast-burning sugars, helping you feel full for longer. All the recipes are tried and tested to be delicious, nutritious and simple to prepare.

Q: DOES THE SORT OF INGREDIENTS YOU BUY MAKE A DIFFERENCE?

A: The recipes in this book include as many 'whole' foods as possible. Whole foods are those tasty delights that are either completely free from refinement or processing, or those that have been meddled with as little as possible. Buying quality ingredients will help support your health and ensure you are getting the maximum goodness from your food.

Food ethics is also something I feel strongly about. I always do my very best to ensure animal welfare is at the forefront of my mind when I shop for food. I believe that free-range and organic animal products are the best options, both for the animal's welfare and our own health. While I understand these products cost a little more, I firmly believe they should be considered when buying your ingredients.

Q: ARE THE RECIPES EXPENSIVE?

A: Prepping your food and being organised can actually help cut your food bill. If you want to buy organic and free-range – something I'd encourage you to do if you can – it might be a little bit more expensive. Thankfully, there are ways you can keep the costs down when you're shopping for this plan. I'll touch upon preparing your meals in bulk later on the next page, and the same can be done when you're buying. Buy frozen fruit and veg where possible so you can use the quantities you need without anything going to waste, and I'd also suggest giving your local greengrocer or butcher a try as you might be able to get a deal – and you'll also be helping your local independent shopkeepers at the same time.

Q: I WORK IN AN OFFICE AND WILL OFTEN HAVE BREAKFAST AND LUNCH THERE. WHAT DO I DO?

A: This is where being organised about your meals comes into play. Benjamin Franklin famously said, 'By failing to prepare, you are preparing to fail.' Regardless of which menu you're choosing from and whether you have your meals at work or at home, I would recommend that you:

- Bulk-buy ingredients to save money and time.
- Cook several meals at a time. Cooking in bulk and separating them into portions will save you so much time (and washing up).
- Invest in some Tupperware or other sealable boxes and a cooler bag.
- Stay organised. Not just in your first week, but EVERY week. It will soon become second nature. If you work all week, decide at the weekend what meals you'll be eating and organise your food shop accordingly so you have all the right ingredients. Then, if possible, bulk-prepare and freeze extra portions on the Sunday night so you've got something you can grab easily when you come in tired from work during the week.

Some of the simpler lunches can also be prepped at work if you take the ingredients with you.

Q: I'M A VEGETARIAN. ARE THERE RECIPES IN THE BOOK I CAN USE?

A: A lot of the recipes for breakfast and snacks are vegetarian-friendly, but the recipes in the book haven't been designed specifically for a veggie diet. However, over recent years I have worked with more and more vegetarians and it has been a huge trend in fitness, so I do want to give you substitutes for the most used meats in this book so you can follow the recipes too – see table overleaf. N.B. These substitutes have been picked to match the calories as closely as possible. As a result the macros, especially the protein levels, may not match the 20/40/40 set-up.

If you would like a more accurate menu as a vegetarian in terms of macros then I offer a monthly nutrition plan on my website that provides full calculated vegetarian recipes every month.

Original ingredient	Veggie alternative	Directions
Chicken	Quorn chicken	To match the calories, multiply the chicken weight by 1.2. You could use tempeh instead, which is a slightly better match in terms of protein. However, you would need to multiply the original chicken weight by 0.65, so quantities might be a bit small.
Salmon steaks or smoked salmon	firm tofu	This has a pretty good protein/fat balance. Multiply the amount of salmon by 1.25 to get the right quantity.
Tinned tuna	tempeh	Tempeh is high in protein for a vegetarian food, but because it contains some fat and carbs you'll need to multiply by 0.65 to match the calorie content. Alternatively, you can use Quorn mince as a 1:1 swap, but your dishes will taste quite different.
Sirloin steak	Quorn sausages	This has a 1:1 calorific match so you can use the same number of grams. There'll just be a few extra carbs, but not many.
Rump steak	Quorn steak	This has a 1:1 calorific match so you can use the same number of grams. An alternative is tempeh – multiply the weight of the rump steak by 0.75.

Q: DO I HAVE TO EAT THE RECIPES IN THIS BOOK, OR CAN I EAT WHAT I LIKE SO LONG AS I'M STICKING TO MY CALORIE BUDGET?

A: You could, but I would encourage you to follow the recipes in the book exactly. It will be the easiest way to ensure you are consuming the right calories and will make it easier to track and monitor progress.

Q: CAN I EAT OUT?

A: My first tip to get the results you want would always be to follow the food plan exactly, but there's more to life than that: most of us love eating out with family and friends from time to time. I'd suggest trying to avoid eating out frequently as, in reality, when we eat out, we tend to consume more calories. We eat the nibbles at the table, we try each other's food and we snack on things without realising it. Also, the menus will likely have foods that will tempt us away from our plan.

So how do we navigate these mealtime challenges? Be aware of your daily calories. It might sound boring, but it's part of the process of achieving results. No one said looking and feeling amazing was easy! Let's not forget that you're on the plan for your own benefit. If you're choosing the restaurant or you know where you're going, you could look at the menu in advance and see if there's an option that fits your plan. Find an option as close as possible to the meal you'd be eating if you were staying in. It won't be a perfect match, but the closer you can get, the better. If you can't find something suitable, then ask if they can cook something that suits the plan more exactly. Most restaurants, in my experience, will, if asked courteously, cook something specifically for you that meets your requirements. They'll have the ingredients and the chef will have the skills, so there's no harm in asking. If all else fails, then you could try balancing the rest of your daily calories to fit the meal in. If this means eating less during the other meals in that day, then so be it. Just aim to get your daily calories correct, as best you can.

Q: CAN I HAVE A CHEAT DAY EVERY NOW AND THEN?

A: A cheat day is a planned date when you break the diet and eat what you want, the idea being that you will be 'good' for longer if you allow yourself the occasional guilt-free 'bad' day. The theory is one thing but the reality can be different; cheat days often turn to cheat weekends, which turn to cheat weeks which turn to cheat months . . . you get the picture. Naturally over the eight-week duration of this plan there will be moments you want to eat something not from the menu. I would suggest you still play it smart as you can easily ruin a week's hard work in one day of overeating. Once you are at a weight/bodyfat level you are happy with you can include more flexible meals, but just be careful not to fall into bad habits.

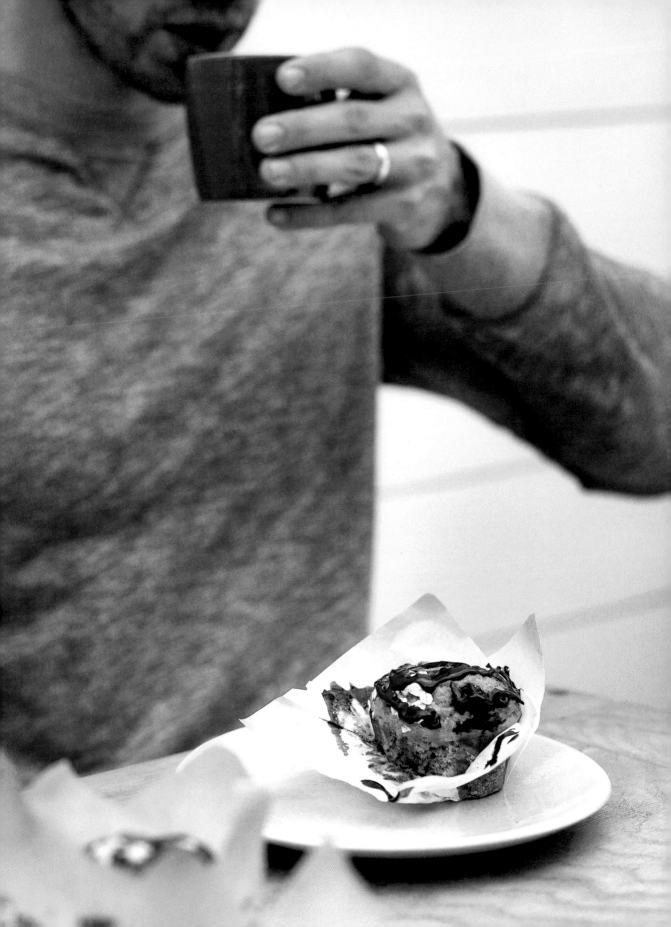

Q: CAN I DRINK ALCOHOL ON THE PLAN?

A: Let me be straight with you. During this plan, I want to discourage alcohol intake. I know. We all like a drink now and again, but I want you to succeed more than I want you to have a drink. By the end of the plan you will have absolutely earned one, I have no doubt about that, but while you're in the process of creating your incredible physique, let's try to give it a miss. Before you slam this book shut in a fit of alcohol-starved rage, give the box below a read – I promise you there are some very real reasons why alcohol will derail your progress.

REASONS TO AVOID ALCOHOL … AT LEAST FOR THE NEXT EIGHT WEEKS!

1. Alcohol has calories

When you're working out your calorie intake, alcohol is often overlooked. If it's something you've glossed over in the past, then you should be aware that alcohol supplies almost twice as many calories as equivalent amounts of protein and carbohydrates. Alcohol might not have any fat, but it does have an energy value, often in the shape of carbs. This comes from the fruit used in the creation of wine, or from the wheat, hops and barley used to brew beer. Even spirits aren't without sugar, thanks to the carbonated mixers they often come with. Alcohol works out about 7 calories per gram, only 2 less than fat. Alcohol also doesn't have any nutritional benefits, so all those calories you could have used on a tasty, nutritious meal are effectively wasted.

2. Alcohol increases appetite

From a scientific point of view you eat more when you've been drinking because the alcohol excites the neurons that incite hunger. In addition, alcohol has a way of relaxing our thoughts enough to do things we probably shouldn't and eat things we almost definitely shouldn't. Those foods will often come covered in grease (a.k.a. fat), salt, creamy sauces or often all of them at once. Collectively, these will become a recipe for excessive calorie intake, enough to throw your plan into a tailspin.

3. Alcohol reduces your chances of losing weight over time

Alcohol is an irritant to the lining of your stomach, gradually weakening your liver and kidneys.

As the lining is weakened, so the food you eat is digested less efficiently. This affects your metabolism and, as a consequence, negatively impacts your efforts to lose weight.

4. Alcohol can lower testosterone levels

Testosterone levels can be lowered if you drink alcohol regularly, especially among men. These lower levels have a direct impact on the ability to both burn fat and contribute to lean muscle mass.

5. Alcohol and the fat battle

As seen above, drinking alcohol can easily push you over your calorie budget for the day. This may cause some of the calories from the food you have eaten to be stored as body fat. In addition, alcohol disrupts your fat-burning potential and may drastically decrease fat burning for hours after drinking.

Q: I'VE DIETED BEFORE AND FOUND IT HARD TO KEEP THE WEIGHT OFF. AM I GOING TO STRUGGLE?

A: The real issue is that for those who have previously lost and gained significant weight, their 'energy out' will potentially be slightly lower than for people who were always lean. Losing weight, or more specifically losing it and keeping it off, is going to be accompanied by adaptive responses. Someone who has gained weight and dieted will often need fewer calories each day than someone who has always been the same weight. The more frequently you have dieted in the past and the more extreme the regime, the greater the chance that your body will have become more sensitive. This doesn't mean that you have ruined your metabolism and cannot lose weight. It simply means you may require slightly fewer calories than you might expect.

If you have dieted before, successfully or otherwise, you can still achieve results with this plan. If you follow the plan based on your current information you will make good progress. If you find yourself not dropping weight quickly enough or not at all then we can re-evaluate your calorie needs – see 'Meeting Your Expectations', page 257.

THE RECIPES

Over the next pages you'll find a selection of delicious breakfasts, lunches, dinners and snacks.

You'll notice that the grams for each ingredient are very specific. This is because, to ensure you are eating the optimum number of calories each day, the recipes have been calculated. You will see by looking at the various calorie options how just a few grams here and few grams there can add up and potentially take you into the next calorie category. When weighing your food, therefore, try to keep it as accurate as possible, but if there are slight ups and downs in your measuring don't stress. These will average out over the duration of your plan.

Some of the ingredients are given as teaspoons or tablespoons. I would recommend you use a measuring spoon for accuracy. A teaspoon should be 5ml, and tablespoon 15ml. Not using a measuring spoon can make a significant difference. For example, a measured tablespoon of peanut butter weighs about 16g and contains under 100 calories; a rounded tablespoon of peanut butter can easily weight up to 40g, and contain well over 200 calories.

The calorie and macro content of the recipes have been calculated using official national statistics data. There will always be some minor variation between products produced by different companies, or natural variation in basic produce. However, the differences between calculated and actual caloric content when you prepare a meal or snack will be minor, and will average out in the long run.

All the recipes serve one, but I encourage you to double or triple the measurements where relevant so you can freeze/save the other portions for another day.

For recipes containing whey protein, you can get my recommendations here: www.davidkingsbury.co.uk/supplements.

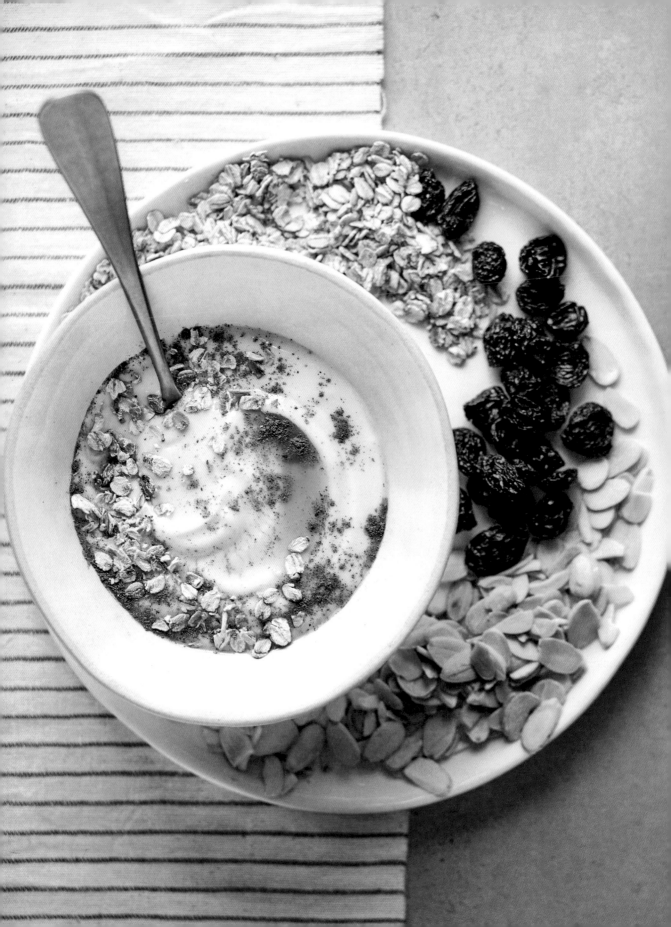

CINNAMON AND NUT OATS WITH NATURAL YOGURT

I absolutely love cinnamon. I add it to almost every meal! It isn't just because I love the taste; cinnamon also has the impressive ability to help regulate blood sugar. This is one of my go-to recipes for a quick, easy and delicious breakfast.

1. Place the oats and the flaked almonds under a medium-hot grill and lightly toast until just brown.

2. Meanwhile, mix the protein powder, yogurt, maple syrup and cinnamon together, using a blender or mixer if necessary.

3. Add the toasted oats, raisins and almonds and enjoy.

note: Skyr can be substituted for any Greek fat-free yogurt and you can use flavoured or unflavoured whey protein (you can find good quality whey on my website).

INGREDIENTS	1	2	3	4	5	6
Rolled oats	1 tbsp	1 tbsp	1.5 tbsp	2 tbsp	2 tbsp	2.5 tbsp
Flaked almonds	21 g	28 g	35 g	42 g	49 g	56 g
Whey protein	18 g	24 g	30 g	36 g	42 g	48 g
Skyr Natural Yogurt	60 g	80 g	100 g	120 g	140 g	160 g
Maple syrup	0.5 tsp	0.5 tsp	0.5 tsp	0.5 tsp	0.5 tsp	1 tsp
Ground cinnamon	0.5 tsp	1 tsp	1 tsp	1 tsp	1.5 tsp	1.5 tsp
Raisins	6 g	8 g	10 g	12 g	14 g	16 g

RASPBERRY CHIA PUDDING

Chia seeds are packed with fibre, protein and nutrients. They add great texture to this dish and are nice and filling even though they are actually low in carbs. Give this recipe a go for a simple and satisfying breakfast. You need to prepare it the night before.

1. Blend the almond milk, yogurt, honey and raspberries, saving a few of the best raspberries for topping.

2. Stir in the whey protein and chia seeds and pour into a sealed jar or Tupperware container.

3. Leave in a fridge overnight, allowing the chia seeds to expand in the liquid.

4. Serve with a topping of the saved raspberries.

INGREDIENTS	1	2	3	4	5	6
Almond milk, unsweetened	180 ml	240 ml	300 ml	360 ml	420 ml	480 ml
Greek yogurt, 0% fat	60 g	80 g	100 g	120 g	140 g	160 g
Honey	0.5 tsp	0.5 tsp	0.5 tsp	1 tsp	1 tsp	1 tsp
Raspberries	48 g	64 g	80 g	96 g	112 g	128 g
Whey protein	19 g	26 g	32 g	38 g	45 g	51 g
Chia seeds	27 g	36 g	45 g	54 g	63 g	72 g

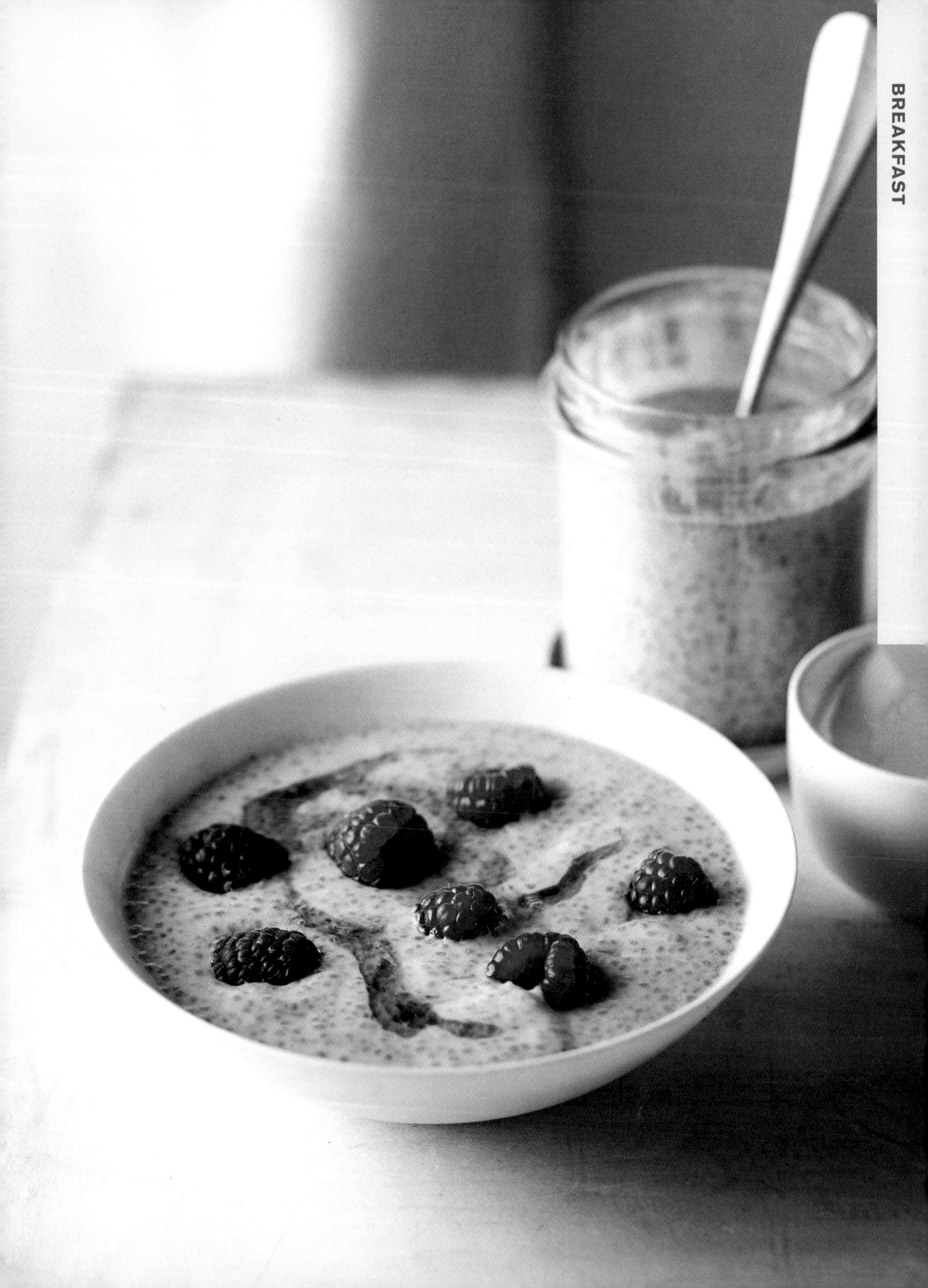

BERRY AND DARK CHOCOLATE PROTEIN PORRIDGE

This sounds great and it tastes as good as it sounds. You may ask how it can hit your macros. Don't worry: I've got it covered . . . in chocolate!

1. Put the chia, flax and coconut in a blender with the milk and protein powder and blend to a paste.

2. Add the oats and cook in a pan on a medium heat for 1–2 minutes to thicken, stirring occasionally.

3. Pour in the raspberries and blueberries and warm through for a further minute.

4. Finally, finely chop the dark chocolate and stir it into the porridge so it has just melted into streaks but not mixed in completely. Serve immediately.

note: You can use flavoured or unflavoured whey protein (you can find good quality whey on my website).

INGREDIENTS	1	2	3	4	5	6
Chia seeds	0.5 tbsp	1 tbsp	1 tbsp	1 tbsp	1.5 tbsp	1.5 tbsp
Flax seeds	0.5 tbsp	1 tbsp	1 tbsp	1 tbsp	1.5 tbsp	1.5 tbsp
Desiccated coconut	0.5 tbsp	1 tbsp	1 tbsp	1 tbsp	1.5 tbsp	1.5 tbsp
Milk, semi-skimmed	96 ml	128 ml	160 ml	192 ml	224 ml	256 ml
Whey protein	24 g	32 g	40 g	48 g	56 g	64 g
Oats	1 tbsp	1.5 tbsp	2 tbsp	2.5 tbsp	3 tbsp	3 tbsp
Raspberries	11 g	15 g	19 g	23 g	27 g	30 g
Blueberries	6 g	8 g	10 g	12 g	14 g	16 g
Dark chocolate (70–85% cocoa)	12 g	16 g	20 g	24 g	28 g	32 g

BANANA AND CINNAMON PORRIDGE

Who knew that a low-carb porridge would taste so good? This is a great warming breakfast that is seriously good. Nothing beats the flavour of sweet banana with the great texture of the seeds and coconut plus that delicious dash of cinnamon.

1. Blend the flax seeds, chia seeds and coconut to a fine powder. Add the whey protein and almond milk, blend again and pour into a pan.

2. Cook on a low to medium heat until the porridge has thickened, stirring occasionally. Don't allow it to bubble vigorously.

3. Add the cinnamon and sliced banana and stir through before serving.

note: You can use flavoured or unflavoured whey protein (you can find good quality whey on my website).

INGREDIENTS	1	2	3	4	5	6
Flax seeds	1 tbsp	1.5 tbsp	2 tbsp	2.5 tbsp	3 tbsp	3 tbsp
Chia seeds	0.5 tbsp	1 tbsp	1 tbsp	1 tbsp	1.5 tbsp	1.5 tbsp
Desiccated coconut	0.5 tbsp	1 tbsp	1 tbsp	1 tbsp	1.5 tbsp	1.5 tbsp
Whey protein	30 g	40 g	50 g	60 g	70 g	80 g
Almond milk, unsweetened	90 ml	120 ml	150 ml	180 ml	210 ml	240 ml
Ground cinnamon	0.5 tsp	1 tsp	1 tsp	1 tsp	1.5 tsp	1.5 tsp
Banana	51 g	68 g	85 g	102 g	119 g	136 g

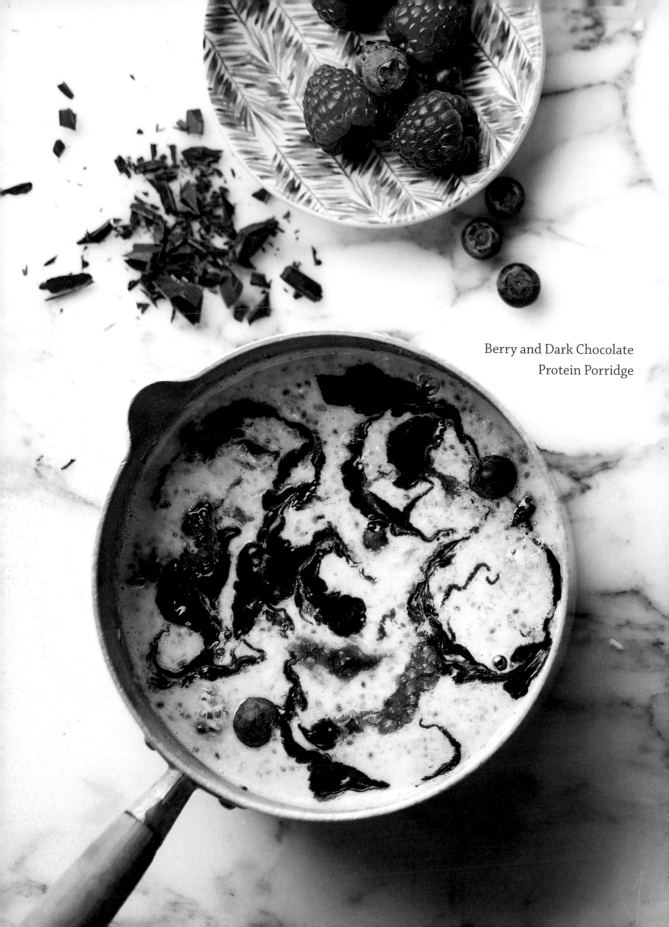

Berry and Dark Chocolate
Protein Porridge

Banana and Cinnamon Porridge

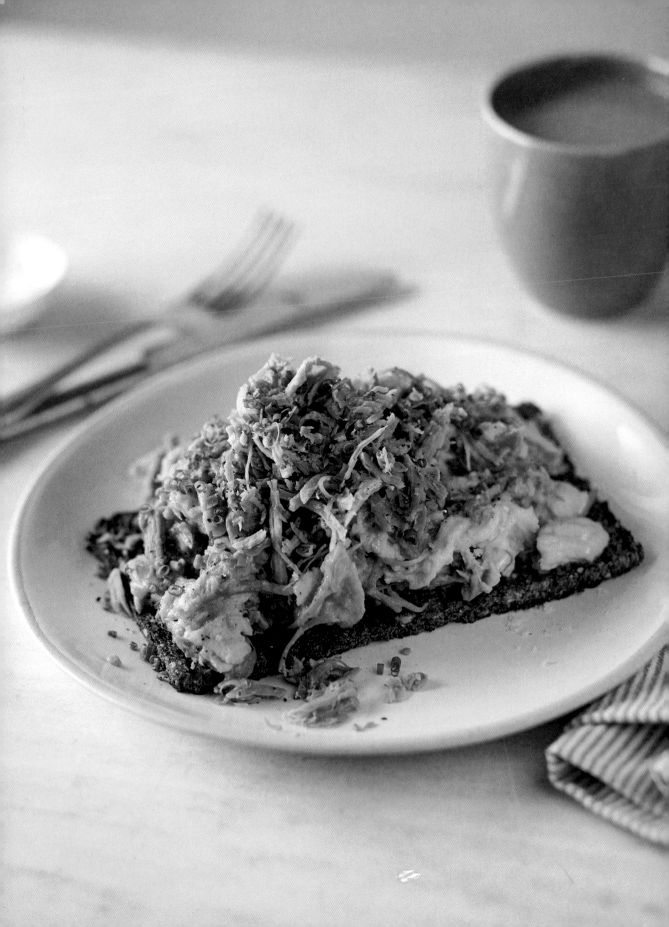

EGG AND HAM ON RYE

Eggs are one of my favourite things to eat and are packed full of protein; this meal is quick and easy to cook so it can easily fit into a busy lifestyle. I enjoy my rye bread best when it is well toasted.

1. Scramble the eggs in a pan over a medium heat, stirring in the chopped ham and chives.

2. Toast the bread and butter it. Serve with the eggs.

note: slices of bread assume you are using a standard pre-sliced loaf of rye bread. If you are using dense 'pumpernickel' rye bread, use the weights given in brackets rather than slices.

INGREDIENTS	1	2	3	4	5	6
Eggs	2 small	3 small	3 medium	4 small	5 small	6 small
Deli ham, chopped	72 g	96 g	120 g	144 g	168 g	192 g
Chives, finely chopped	0.5 tbsp	1 tbsp	1 tbsp	1 tbsp	1.5 tbsp	1.5 tbsp
Rye bread	1 slice (36 g)	1½ slices (48 g)	1½ slices (60 g)	2 slices (72 g)	2 slices (84 g)	2½ slices (96 g)
Salted butter	0.5 tsp	0.5 tsp	0.5 tsp	0.5 tsp	0.5 tsp	1 tsp

RASPBERRY ALMOND PANCAKES

Amazing pancakes for a fat-loss recipe? With calories and macros spot-on for your goals? Is this real life? No need to wait for Pancake Day this year. Try this amazing high-protein spin on pancakes.

1. Blend the eggs and egg whites, two-thirds of the raspberries, oat bran and whey protein until the mixture achieves a thick yet still runny consistency.

2. Heat the coconut oil in a large frying pan on a medium heat, and pour in enough batter mixture to make three small pancakes (you might need to do this in batches if you are using the larger quantities).

3. Cook for about 3–5 minutes until the pancakes are holding together, flip and cook for a further 3 minutes on the other side.

4. While the pancakes are cooking, mix a dash of water with the reserved raspberries and cook them in a pan on a low heat, to make a raspberry stew.

5. Serve the pancakes as a stack, with the stewed raspberry in between the layers and flaked almonds sprinkled on top.

note: You can use flavoured or unflavoured whey protein (you can find good quality whey on my website).

INGREDIENTS	1	2	3	4	5	6
Eggs	1 small	1 small	1 medium	1 large	2 small	2 small
Egg white	1 small	1 small	1 medium	1 large	2 small	2 small
Raspberries	84 g	112 g	140 g	168 g	196 g	224 g
Oat bran	18 g	24 g	30 g	36 g	42 g	48 g
Whey protein	21 g	28 g	35 g	42 g	49 g	56 g
Coconut oil	0.5 tsp	0.5 tsp	0.5 tsp	0.5 tsp	0.5 tsp	1 tsp
Flaked almonds	12 g	16 g	20 g	24 g	28 g	32 g

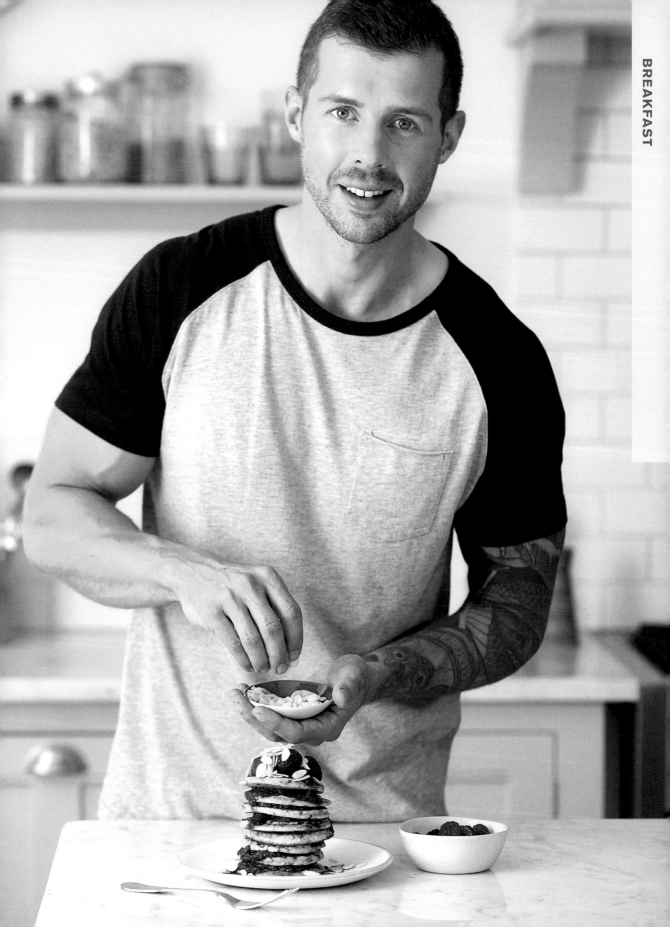

HUEVOS RANCHEROS

This is a solid weekend recipe for me and the tomato steak base is great to cook in bulk so as to make a few days' worth in one go. It is absolutely packed full of flavour and worth every second of the cooking time.

1. Cook the onions in a non-stick pan over a gentle heat for 3–4 minutes until they are lightly browned, then add the red pepper, red chilli, garlic and beef steak, cut into strips. Fry for a further 5 minutes.

2. Mash the tinned tomatoes with the back of a fork to break them up and add to the pan with the drained black beans and bay leaves. Stir through while bringing to the boil then simmer for 8 minutes to reduce the mixture.

3. Make a small well in the tomato mix for each egg and break one into each well. Cover the pan with a lid and cook for a further 4 minutes to set the eggs.

4. Meanwhile, make the tortilla pancake by mixing together the yogurt, ground almonds, baking powder, chilli powder and egg.

5. Pour the batter into a hot pan and cook until each side is golden, flipping halfway. Serve onto a plate. Layer over sliced tomato.

6. Pour over the tomato, steak and egg mix from the pan and season to taste.

INGREDIENTS	1	2	3	4	5	6
For the tomato and bean mixture						
Onion, chopped	18 g	24 g	30 g	36 g	42 g	48 g
Red pepper, diced	36 g	48 g	60 g	72 g	84 g	96 g
Red chilli pepper, finely chopped	6 g	8 g	10 g	12 g	14 g	16 g
Garlic, crushed	0.5 clove	0.5 clove	0.5 clove	0.5 clove	0.5 clove	1 clove
Beef steak	42 g	56 g	70 g	84 g	98 g	112 g
Tomato, tinned	90 g	120 g	150 g	180 g	210 g	240 g
Black beans, tinned	36 g	48 g	60 g	72 g	84 g	96 g

Bay leaf	2 leaves	2 leaves	3 leaves	4 leaves	4 leaves	5 leaves
Tomato, sliced	51 g	68 g	85 g	102 g	119 g	136 g
Eggs	1 large	2 small	2 medium	3 small	3 medium	3 large
For the tortilla pancake						
Greek yogurt, 0% fat	1 tbsp	1.5 tbsp	2 tbsp	2.5 tbsp	3 tbsp	3 tbsp
Ground almonds	0.5 tbsp	1 tbsp	1 tbsp	1 tbsp	1.5 tbsp	1.5 tbsp
Baking powder	0.5 tsp	0.5 tsp	0.5 tsp	0.5 tsp	0.5 tsp	0.5 tsp
Chilli powder	0.5 tsp	0.5 tsp	0.5 tsp	0.5 tsp	0.5 tsp	0.5 tsp
Eggs	1 small	1 small	1 medium	1 large	2 small	2 small

FRUIT AND YOGURT

This yogurt and fruit breakfast is fresh and easy for a summer morning. High-protein yogurt with nutrient-rich berries and almond butter: it doesn't get much better than this!

1. Mix the protein powder and almond butter with a small amount of the yogurt to make a paste. Slowly add the remaining yogurt while continuing to mix thoroughly.

2. Top with the blueberries and slices of strawberries..

note: Skyr can be substituted for any Greek fat-free yogurt and you can use flavoured or unflavoured whey protein (you can find good quality whey on my website).

INGREDIENTS	1	2	3	4	5	6
Whey protein	12 g	16 g	20 g	24 g	28 g	32 g
Almond butter	24 g	32 g	40 g	48 g	56 g	64 g
Skyr Natural Yogurt	120 g	160 g	200 g	240 g	280 g	320 g
Blueberries	42 g	56 g	70 g	84 g	98 g	112 g
Strawberries, sliced	42 g	56 g	70 g	84 g	98 g	112 g

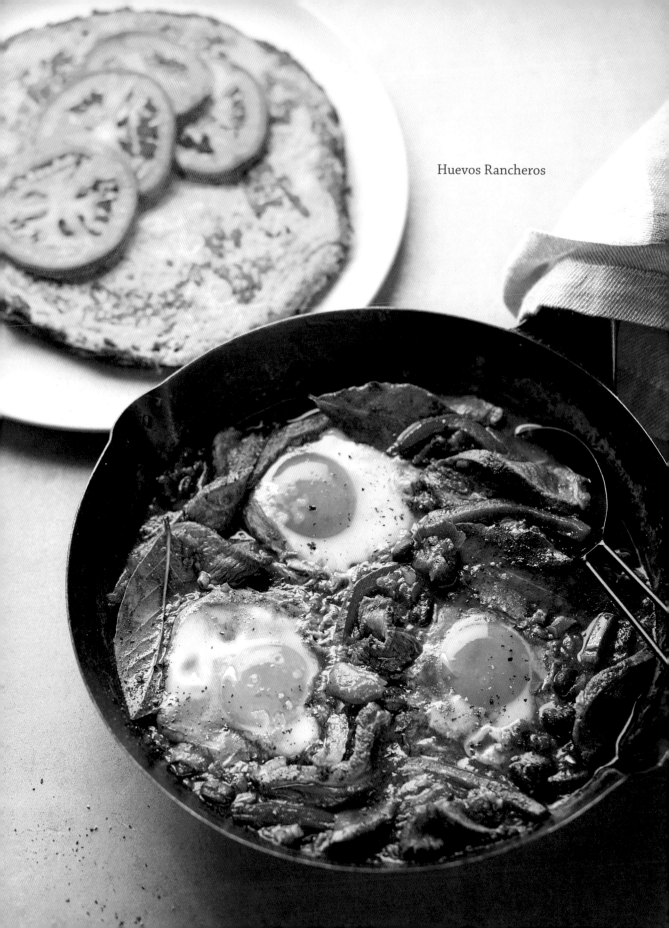

Huevos Rancheros

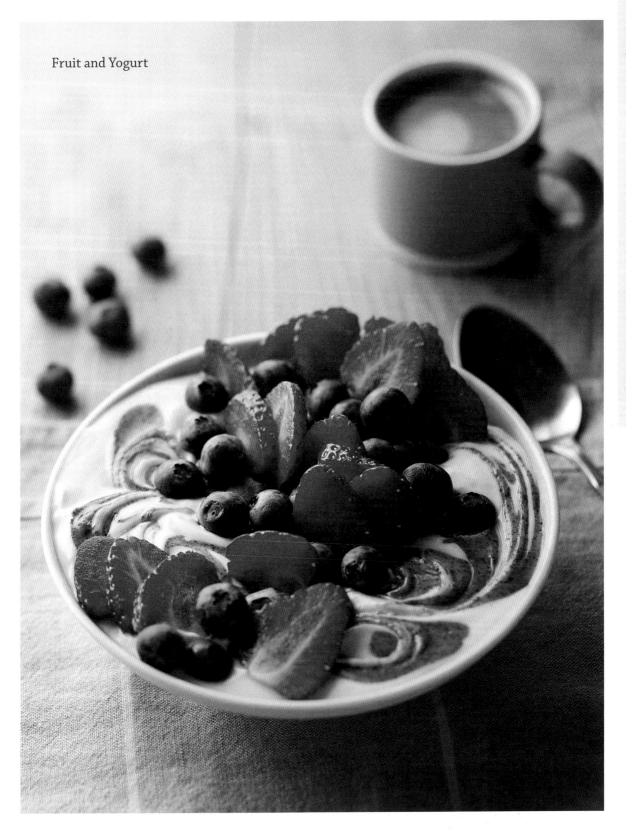

Fruit and Yogurt

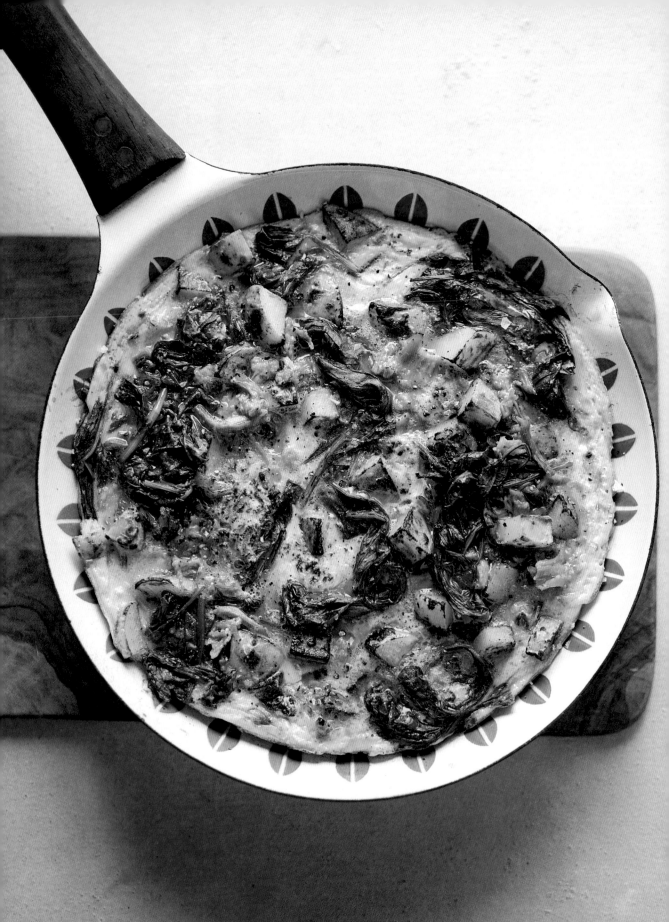

HAM, POTATO, ONION AND SPINACH FRITTATA

What's not to like with this go-to recipe? I absolutely love a frittata any time of day and this breakfast special is right up my street.

1. Pre-heat the grill.

2. Heat the coconut oil over a high heat using a grill-proof pan. Finely chop the onions, then add to the pan and fry until brown.

3. Cube the potatoes into ½ cm chunks, then add to the onions and continue to cook over a medium heat for 5 minutes.

4. Add the spinach and cover (if you don't have a lid you could use foil) until the spinach is fully wilted.

5. Break in the eggs and add in the chopped ham. Give it all a quick stir and leave covered until the base is set, about 5 minutes.

6. Remove the lid and then place the pan under the grill to cook the top of the frittata – about 5–10 minutes depending on your grill and which size dish you're making.

7. When the top of the frittata is fully set, remove from the grill, put onto a plate, garnish with coriander and season to taste.

INGREDIENTS	1	2	3	4	5	6
Coconut oil	0.5 tsp	0.5 tsp	0.5 tsp	0.5 tsp	0.5 tsp	1 tsp
Onions	36 g	48 g	60 g	72 g	84 g	96 g
New potatoes	78 g	104 g	130 g	156 g	182 g	208 g
Baby spinach	36 g	48 g	60 g	72 g	84 g	96 g
Eggs	2 small	3 small	3 medium	4 small	5 small	6 small
Deli ham	78 g	104 g	130 g	156 g	182 g	208 g
Coriander	1 handful	1 handful	1 handful	1 handful	1 handful	1 handful

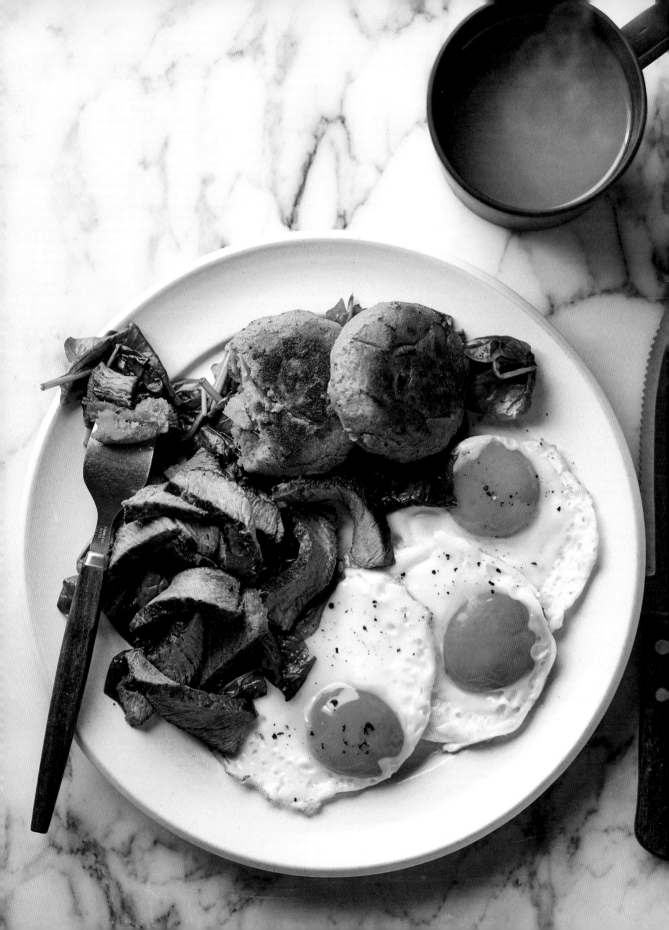

STEAK AND EGGS, WITH SWEET POTATO HASH AND SAUTÉED SPINACH

This is a great hearty breakfast with many of my favourite ingredients combined.

1. Peel and finely dice the sweet potato, then add to a pan of boiling water. Boil until soft, about 10 minutes.

2. Remove half the sweet potato with a slotted spoon and boil the rest until it's really soft, a further 8 minutes.

3. Drain and mash the softer sweet potato, then stir in the chunks and form the mixture into burger-sized patties using your hands.

4. Heat the oil in a very large pan, adding the patties and steak. Fry the patties until browned on both sides and cook the steak to preference.

5. Break the eggs into the pan and fry for the last 3 minutes of the cooking time, then serve it all onto a plate.

6. Add the spinach to the hot pan and sauté for 2 minutes until it wilts. Add to the plate and season to taste before serving.

INGREDIENTS	1	2	3	4	5	6
Sweet potato	81 g	108 g	135 g	162 g	189 g	216 g
Olive oil	0.5 tsp	1 tsp	1 tsp	1.5 tsp	1.5 tsp	2 tsp
Beef steak, lean	81 g	108 g	135 g	162 g	189 g	216 g
Egg	1 large	2 small	2 medium	3 small	3 medium	3 large
Baby spinach	36 g	48 g	60 g	72 g	84 g	96 g

SCRAMBLED EGG, TURKEY BACON, SPINACH AND RYE

This is my take on a healthy fry-up. Easily cooked in under 10 minutes, this high-protein great-tasting meal is a real winner.

1. Heat a frying pan on the hob, lay the turkey rashers in and cook them on both sides until browned.

2. Add the spinach and sauté for a couple of minutes until it has wilted.

3. Meanwhile, break the eggs into another hot pan and scramble with half the butter.

4. Toast the rye bread and spread with the remaining butter.

5. Serve together and season to taste.

note: slices of bread assume you are using a standard pre-sliced loaf of rye bread. If you are using dense 'pumpernickel' rye bread, use the weights given in brackets rather than slices.

INGREDIENTS	1	2	3	4	5	6
Turkey rashers	84 g	113 g	142 g	171 g	201 g	229 g
Baby spinach	48 g	54 g	60 g	66 g	72 g	78 g
Eggs	1 large	2 small	2 medium	3 small	3 medium	3 large
Salted butter	1 tsp	1 tsp	1.5 tsp	1.5 tsp	2 tsp	2 tsp
Rye bread	1 slice (30 g)	1 slice (40 g)	1½ slices (50 g)	1½ slices (60 g)	2 slices (70 g)	2 slices (80 g)

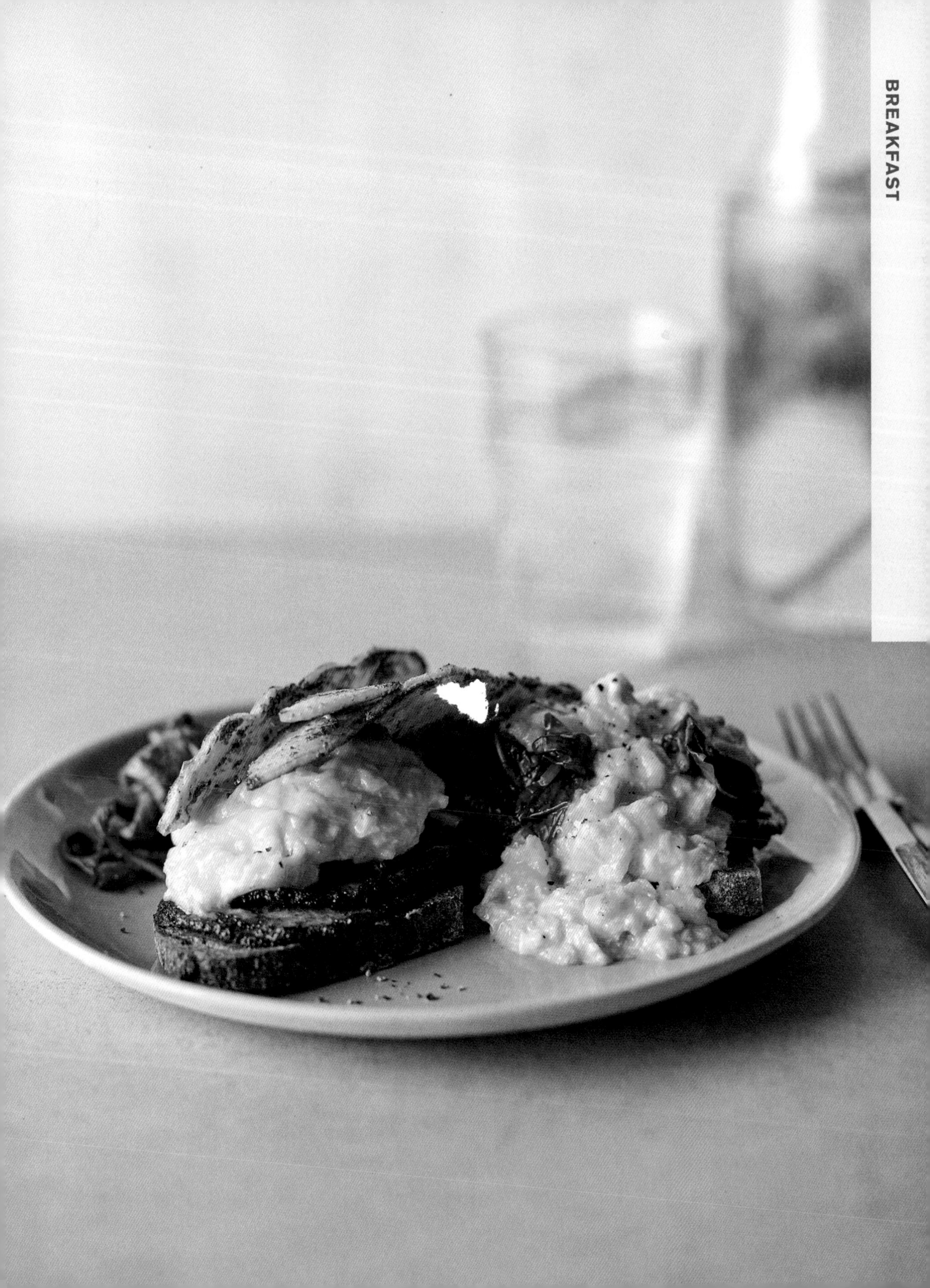

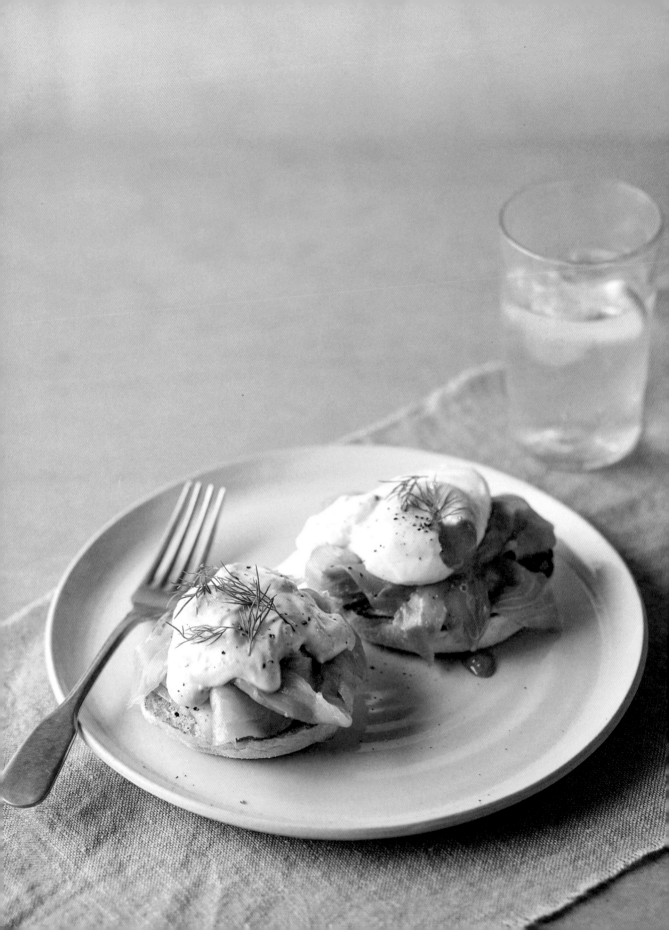

SALMON EGGS ROYALE WITH YOGURT HOLLANDAISE

This is a smoked salmon recipe with eggs cooked in my favourite way. Featuring a modern healthy take on the classic hollandaise sauce, it works a treat. I've given the muffins in both approximate amount and grams – grams are more precise so try to go for this, but amount is easier!

1. Beat together the yogurt, egg yolk and lemon juice in a heatproof bowl. Place the bowl over a small pan of boiling water, so that the base of the bowl does not touch the water.

2. Cook for 15 minutes until thickened, stirring frequently. Carefully remove the bowl from the heat and stir in the mustard and dill.

3. Break the egg(s) into a cup. Heat a pan of water to just under a rolling boil, vigorously stir the water until it creates a vortex and pour the egg(s) into the middle. Poach for 3–4 minutes until the white is set and yolk is still runny.

4. Meanwhile, toast the muffin and lay the smoked salmon on top. Remove the egg from the pan with a slotted spoon and add to the plate, pouring the yogurt hollandaise on top. Season to taste.

INGREDIENTS	1	2	3	4	5	6
Greek yogurt, 0% fat	51 g	68 g	85 g	102 g	119 g	136 g
Egg yolk	1 small	1 small	1 large	1 large	2 small	2 small
Lemon juice	0.5 tsp	1 tsp	1 tsp	1 tsp	1.5 tsp	1.5 tsp
Dijon mustard	0.5 tsp	0.5 tsp	0.5 tsp	0.5 tsp	0.5 tsp	1 tsp
Dill, finely chopped	0.5 tsp	0.5 tsp	0.5 tsp	0.5 tsp	0.5 tsp	1 tsp
Egg	1 small	1 small	1 large	1 large	2 small	2 small
English muffin	½ (30 g)	½ (40 g)	1½ (50 g)	1½ (60 g)	2 (70 g)	2 (80 g)
Smoked salmon	60 g	80 g	100 g	120 g	140 g	160 g

BANANA, CHOCOLATE AND CASHEW SMOOTHIE

This is a really decadent breakfast, but it isn't just a treat. This smoothie is balanced to hit your calories and macros and it seriously delivers on flavour too!

1. Blend all the ingredients together.

2. Check the consistency – if you like your smoothies a little looser then add more water.

3. Enjoy!

note: Skyr can be substituted for any Greek fat-free yogurt and you can use flavoured or unflavoured whey protein (you can find good quality whey on my website).

INGREDIENTS	1	2	3	4	5	6
Almond milk, unsweetened	90 ml	120 ml	150 ml	180 ml	210 ml	240 ml
Skyr Natural Yogurt	48 g	64 g	80 g	96 g	112 g	128 g
Banana, frozen	36 g	48 g	60 g	72 g	84 g	96 g
Whey protein	24 g	32 g	40 g	48 g	56 g	64 g
Cashew nut butter	17 g	22 g	28 g	34 g	39 g	45 g
Cocoa powder	1 tsp	1.5 tsp	2 tsp	2.5 tsp	3 tsp	3 tsp

BERRY AND NUT SMOOTHIE

Berries are high in antioxidants and fibre and have a much lower sugar content than some other fruit. I often add berries to my smoothies to add a delicious fresh flavour. This is a quick and easy smoothie that tastes great.

1. Blend all the ingredients together.

2. Check the consistency – if you like your smoothies a little looser then add more water.

3. Enjoy!

note: Skyr can be substituted for any Greek fat-free yogurt and you can use flavoured or unflavoured whey protein (you can find good quality whey on my website).

INGREDIENTS	1	2	3	4	5	6
Oat milk, unsweetened	120 g	160 g	200 g	240 g	280 g	320 g
Skyr Natural Yogurt	24 g	32 g	40 g	48 g	56 g	64 g
Whey protein	24 g	32 g	40 g	48 g	56 g	64 g
Blackberries	24 g	32 g	40 g	48 g	56 g	64 g
Raspberries	24 g	32 g	40 g	48 g	56 g	64 g
Peanut butter	21 g	28 g	35 g	42 g	49 g	56 g

TURKEY, BACON, SPINACH AND SWEET POTATO QUICHE

Quiches can sometimes seem a bit boring and bland, but this one offers a whole new taste sensation. The sweet potato works better than pastry. No joke!

1. Preheat the oven to 200°C/fan 180°C/gas mark 6.

2. Peel and thinly slice the sweet potato. The slices should be thin enough to bend.

3. Lay the slices in the bottom and up the sides of a non-stick flan dish to make the quiche base. You will need a 15cm dish for the smaller sizes, 20cm for the middle sizes and 25cm for the largest. The slices will shrink, so overlap them well and place several up the sides of the dish. Drizzle over a little of the olive oil, season and bake blind in the oven for 15–20 minutes until very soft.

4. Meanwhile, fry the onion and garlic in the rest of the oil until lightly browned, about 4 minutes, then add the spinach and wilt for 2–3 minutes.

5. Cube the turkey and bacon and fry, in a separate pan, until browned. Spread over the sweet potato base when ready.

6. Whisk the egg with a fork in a cup, then pour over the rest of the quiche ingredients. Turn the oven down to 190C and bake for 35–40 minutes, until the eggs are set

7. Allow to cool, serve still warm or cool

INGREDIENTS	1	2	3	4	5	6
Sweet potato	66 g	88 g	110 g	132 g	154 g	176 g
Olive oil	0.5 tsp	0.5 tsp	0.5 tsp	0.5 tsp	0.5 tsp	1 tsp
Onion, sliced	18 g	24 g	30 g	36 g	42 g	48 g

Garlic, crushed	0.5 clove	1 clove	1 clove	1 clove	1.5 clove	1.5 clove
Baby spinach	24 g	32 g	40 g	48 g	56 g	64 g
Eggs	1 large	2 small	2 medium	3 small	3 medium	3 large
Turkey, diced	60 g	80 g	100 g	120 g	140 g	160 g
Bacon, diced	30 g	40 g	50 g	60 g	70 g	80 g
Chives, finely chopped	1 tbsp	1.5 tbsp	2 tbsp	2.5 tbsp	3 tbsp	3 tbsp

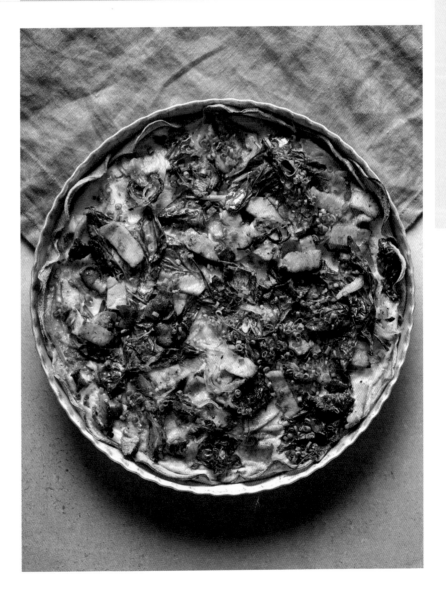

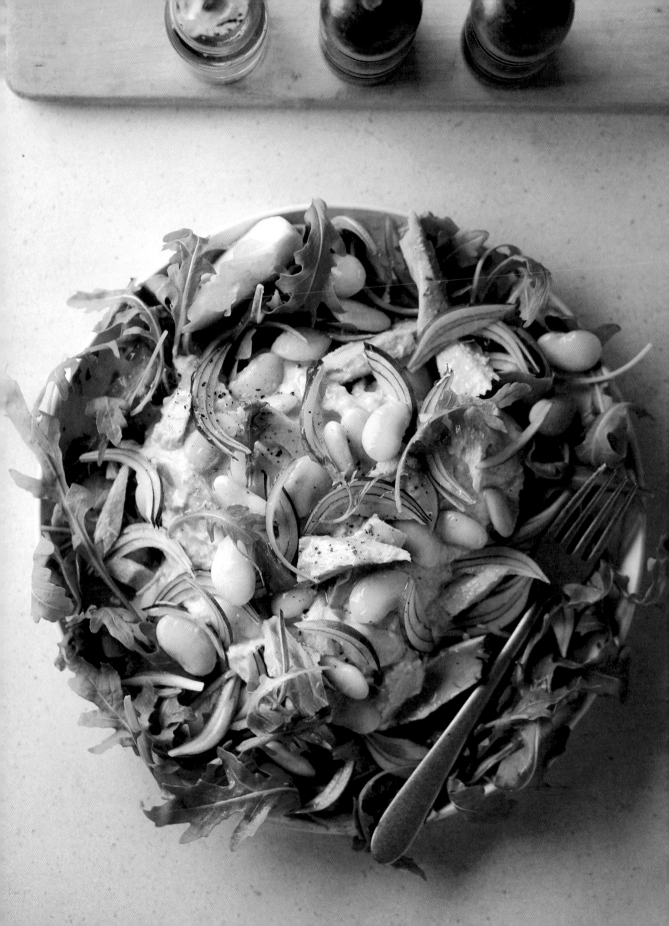

TUNA BEAN SALAD

This lovely fresh-tasting salad with a classic combination of ingredients is possible to whip up in a matter of minutes, making this a great option if time is limited.

1. Mash the avocado and mix in with the Greek yogurt, red onion, lemon juice and garlic.

2. Stir in the tuna and drained butter beans, and serve with rocket drizzled with olive oil.

INGREDIENTS	1	2	3	4	5	6
Avocado	54 g	72 g	90 g	108 g	126 g	144 g
Greek yogurt, 0% fat	48 g	64 g	80 g	96 g	112 g	128 g
Red onion, finely sliced	18 g	24 g	30 g	36 g	42 g	48 g
Lemon juice	1 tsp	1.5 tsp	2 tsp	2.5 tsp	3 tsp	3 tsp
Garlic, crushed	1 clove	1 clove	1 clove	1 clove	1 clove	2 cloves
Tuna, tinned	84 g	112 g	140 g	168 g	196 g	224 g
Butter beans	66 g	88 g	110 g	132 g	154 g	176 g
Rocket leaves	60 g	80 g	100 g	120 g	140 g	160 g
Olive oil	0.5 tsp	0.5 tsp	0.5 tsp	0.5 tsp	0.5 tsp	1 tsp

MEXICAN SPICE BOWL

Time to spice up your life with this bowl of loveliness. It's a great meal to warm you up on a cold winter's day or if you just like food with a bit of a kick.

1. Heat the oil in a pan and add the onion, paprika and chilli powder. Fry on a medium heat until the onions have lightly browned, about 4 minutes.

2. Add the beef mince and fry for another 3–4 minutes to brown slightly, then add the sliced mushrooms, beans and tinned tomatoes.

3. Bring the mixture to the boil then lower to a simmer. Leave uncovered to reduce down for 10–15 minutes.

4. Serve in a bowl with the sour cream on top, and garnish with coriander if you have any.

note: if you don't like your food too spicy, just add less chilli powder or paprika.

INGREDIENTS	1	2	3	4	5	6
Olive oil	1 tsp	1 tsp	1.5 tsp	2 tsp	2 tsp	2.5 tsp
Onion, sliced	36 g	48 g	60 g	72 g	84 g	96 g
Paprika	1 tsp	1.5 tsp	2 tsp	2.5 tsp	3 tsp	3 tsp
Chilli powder	1 tsp	1.5 tsp	2 tsp	2.5 tsp	3 tsp	3 tsp
Beef mince, extra lean	105 g	140 g	175 g	210 g	245 g	280 g
White mushrooms	42 g	56 g	70 g	84 g	98 g	112 g
Red kidney beans, tinned	48 g	64 g	80 g	96 g	112 g	128 g
Tomatoes, tinned	90 g	120 g	150 g	180 g	210 g	240 g
Sour cream	1 tbsp	1.5 tbsp	2 tbsp	2.5 tbsp	3 tbsp	3 tbsp

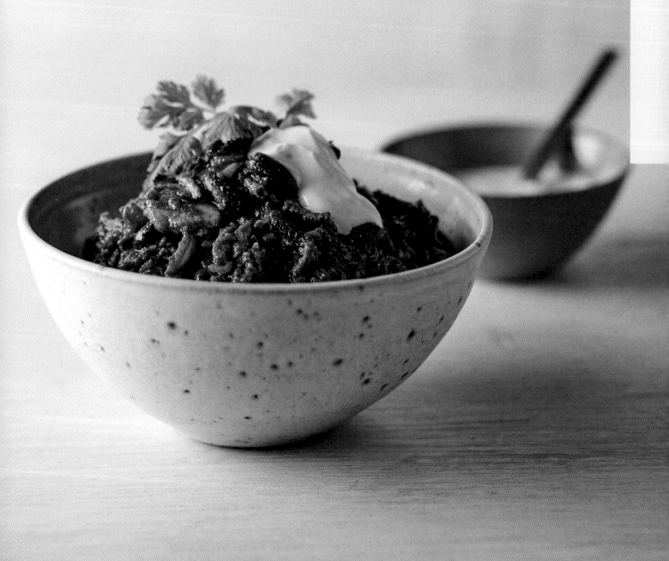

CHIPOTLE CHICKEN WITH BLACK BEAN SALSA

This is a great dish that combines a touch of heat from the jalapeño peppers and a zingy freshness from the lime and coriander. The source of protein is the flavoursome marinated chicken.

1. To make the chipotle mayo: blend together the chipotle peppers in adobo, half the onion, half the coriander and half the juice of the lime. Then mix in the mayonnaise.

2. Place the chicken breasts in a bowl and coat in a third of the mayonnaise mixture, reserving the bulk for serving. Leave to absorb the flavours in a fridge for at least 2 hours.

3. To make the salsa: zest and juice the remainder of the lime and mix with the chopped tomato and jalapeño peppers, drained black beans and olive oil. Finely chop the remaining coriander and onion and add to the salsa.

4. Heat a skillet on high, remove the chicken from the mayonnaise – allowing it to remain well coated – and fry until cooked through, and charred along the skillet ridges, about 6 minutes each side.

5. Serve with the remaining mayo and salsa.

INGREDIENTS	1	2	3	4	5	6
Chipotle peppers in adobo sauce	48 g	64 g	80 g	96 g	112 g	128 g
Onions	18 g	24 g	30 g	36 g	42 g	48 g
Coriander	1 handful	1 handful	1 handful	1 handful	1 handful	1 handful
Lime	0.5 lime	1 lime	1 lime	1 lime	1.5 limes	1.5 limes
Mayonnaise, reduced fat	2.5 tbsp	3 tbsp	4 tbsp	5 tbsp	5.5 tbsp	6.5 tbsp
Chicken breast	102 g	136 g	170 g	204 g	238 g	272 g

Tomatoes, finely chopped	51 g	68 g	85 g	102 g	119 g	136 g
Jalapeño peppers, finely chopped	6 g	8 g	10 g	12 g	14 g	16 g
Black beans, tinned	54 g	72 g	90 g	108 g	126 g	144 g
Olive oil	0.5 tsp	0.5 tsp	0.5 tsp	0.5 tsp	0.5 tsp	1 tsp

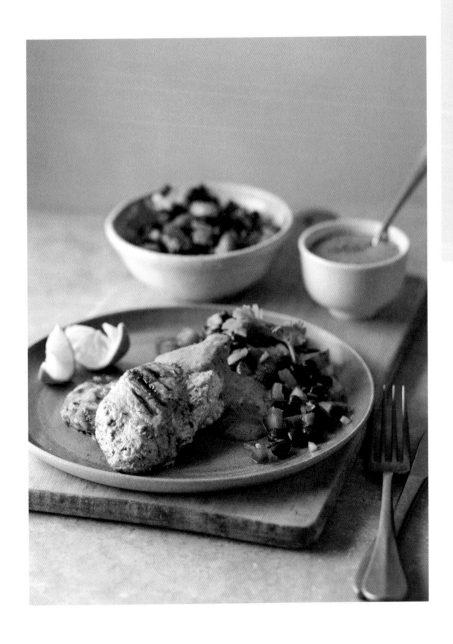

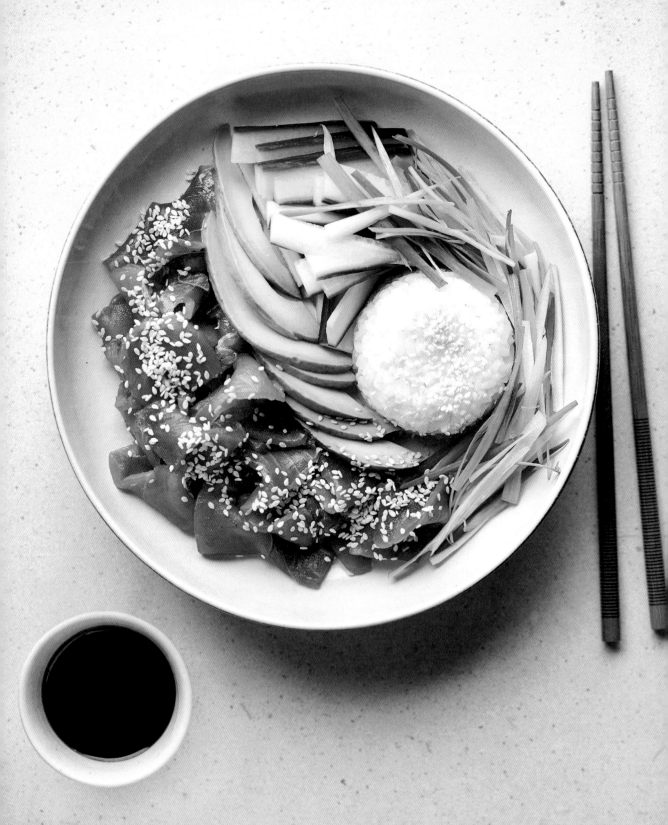

SUSHI BOWL

This sushi bowl is super fresh and packed full of amazing flavour. One of my all time favourites!

1. Rinse sushi rice a few times, sieve, then add vinegar and cold water (2 parts water, 1 part rice). Cover, bring to boil and simmer for 10 minutes, then remove from heat and leave for 15 more minutes with the lid on. Remove from pan and place in a large bowl.

2. Cut tuna, spring onion and cucumber into matchsticks or slices and mix in sesame oil and seeds.

3. Serve veg and tuna over rice, topped with sliced avocado.

note: tuna should be very fresh and you should check with your fishmonger or supermarket that the tuna can be enjoyed raw. If not, it can be cooked in a hot pan before eating.

INGREDIENTS	1	2	3	4	5	6
Sushi rice	15 g	20 g	25 g	30 g	35 g	40 g
Rice vinegar	0.5 tsp	1tsp	1tsp	1tsp	1.5tsp	1.5tsp
Tuna steak	108 g	144 g	180 g	216 g	252 g	288 g
Spring onions	12 g	16 g	20 g	24 g	28 g	32 g
Cucumber	33 g	44 g	55 g	66 g	77 g	88 g
Sesame oil	0.5 tsp	1 tsp	1 tsp	1 tsp	1.5 tsp	1.5 tsp
Sesame seeds	0.5 tbsp	1 tbsp	1 tbsp	1 tbsp	1.5 tbsp	1.5 tbsp
Avocado	24 g	32 g	40 g	48 g	56 g	64 g

CHICKEN, FETA AND SWEET POTATO SALAD

This salad is a real stand-out; the combination of the chicken and sweet potato is something special. The addition of the creamy feta takes it up another level.

1. Peel and dice the sweet potato, place in a pan and cover with water. Bring to the boil and simmer until cooked, about 20 minutes, then drain.

2. Meanwhile, fry the chicken in the oil for 10 minutes, stirring regularly.

3. Add the slices of red pepper and the chilli powder and stir-fry for a further 5 minutes.

4. Remove from the heat and allow to cool.

5. Mix the rocket and cubes of feta cheese in a large bowl. Add the cooled chicken and pepper mix, stir in the sweet potato and drizzle over the lemon juice. Season to taste before serving.

INGREDIENTS	1	2	3	4	5	6
Sweet potato	66 g	88 g	110 g	132 g	154 g	176 g
Chicken breast, sliced	84 g	112 g	140 g	168 g	196 g	224 g
Olive oil	0.5 tsp	1 tsp	1 tsp	1 tsp	1.5 tsp	1.5 tsp
Red pepper, sliced	42 g	56 g	70 g	84 g	98 g	112 g
Chilli powder	0.5 tsp	1 tsp	1 tsp	1 tsp	1.5 tsp	1.5 tsp
Rocket leaves	60 g	80 g	100 g	120 g	140 g	160 g
Feta cheese, cubed	42 g	56 g	70 g	84 g	98 g	112 g
Lemon juice	0.5 tbsp	1 tbsp	1 tbsp	1 tbsp	1.5 tbsp	1.5 tbsp

CHICKEN AND SUN-DRIED TOMATO POTATO SALAD

The combination of the rich flavour of the sun-dried tomatoes with the freshness of the dressing is hard to beat.

1. Bring a pan of water to the boil and add the potato. Boil until soft, about 20 minutes. Drain and cool.

2. Squeeze the excess oil from the sun-dried tomatoes into another pan, then add the chicken and spring onion.

3. Cook, stirring frequently, for 10 minutes, until the chicken is cooked through.

4. In a bowl, mix together the lemon juice, crème fraîche, slices of sun-dried tomato, cooked potato, and the chicken and spring onion.

5. Make a bed of salad leaves and sliced cucumber in a large salad bowl. Pour over the creamy chicken mix and serve.

INGREDIENTS	1	2	3	4	5	6
New potatoes, cut into chunks	75 g	100 g	125 g	150 g	175 g	200 g
Sun-dried tomatoes in oil, sliced	14 g	19 g	24 g	29 g	34 g	38 g
Chicken breast, cut into strips	108 g	144 g	180 g	216 g	252 g	288 g
Spring onions, sliced	12 g	16 g	20 g	24 g	28 g	32 g
Lemon juice	0.5 tsp	1 tsp	1 tsp	1 tsp	1.5 tsp	1.5 tsp
Crème fraîche, half-fat	0.5 tbsp	1 tbsp	1 tbsp	1.5 tbsp	1.5 tbsp	2 tbsp
Mixed salad	45 g	60 g	75 g	90 g	105 g	120 g
Cucumber, sliced	60 g	80 g	100 g	120 g	140 g	160 g

SEITAN 'MEATBALLS' WITH VEG AND TOMATO SAUCE

This great recipe uses seitan – a type of Asian wheat gluten – which is incredibly high in protein. It combines a long list of ingredients, but it's definitely worth the effort for its flavour-packing goodness. I would recommend bulk cooking this, especially the meatballs. They will keep for several months in the freezer.

1. Preheat the oven to 200°C/fan 180°C/gas mark 6.

2. Blend the seitan until smooth, add the pecans and pulse until blended.

3. Empty into a bowl with the breadcrumbs, garlic, parsley, basil, oregano and half the sesame oil. Mix together with your fingertips. Slowly add water until the mixture reaches a sticky consistency that can be shaped easily. Roll the mixture into balls with your hands, about the size of a large strawberry.

4. Place in a baking tray, drizzle over the remaining sesame oil and bake in the oven for 20 mins until browned and slightly crispy, turning halfway through.

5. Meanwhile, chop the pepper, tomatoes and broccoli, fry in half the olive oil, add the chilli powder, tomato puree and oregano, and cook covered for 3–4 minutes.

6. Mix the meatballs when ready into the veg and tomato, drizzle the remainder of the olive oil on top and grate over cheese.

INGREDIENTS	1	2	3	4	5	6
For the seitan 'meatballs'						
Seitan	23 g	30 g	38 g	46 g	53 g	61 g
Pecan nuts	1 pecan	1 pecan	1 pecan	1 pecan	1 pecan	2 pecans
Breadcrumbs	3 g	4 g	5 g	6 g	7 g	8 g
Garlic, crushed	0.5 cloves	0.5 cloves	0.5 cloves	0.5 cloves	0.5 cloves	1 clove
Parsley, finely chopped	0.5 tsp	0.5 tsp	0.5 tsp	0.5 tsp	0.5 tsp	1 tsp
Basil, finely chopped	0.5 tsp	0.5 tsp	0.5 tsp	0.5 tsp	0.5 tsp	1 tsp

Oregano, dried	1 pinch	1 pinch	1 pinch	1 pinch	1 pinch	2 pinches
Sesame oil	0.5 tsp	0.5 tsp	0.5 tsp	0.5 tsp	0.5 tsp	1 tsp
Water	24 ml	32 ml	40 ml	48 ml	56 ml	64 ml
For the veg and tomato sauce						
Red pepper, diced	54 g	72 g	90 g	108 g	126 g	144 g
Tomatoes, diced	42 g	56 g	70 g	84 g	98 g	112 g
Broccoli, cut into small florets	30 g	40 g	50 g	60 g	70 g	80 g
Olive oil	0.5 tbsp	0.5 tbsp	1 tbsp	1 tbsp	1 tbsp	1.5 tbsp
Chilli powder	0.5 tsp	0.5 tsp	0.5 tsp	0.5 tsp	0.5 tsp	1 tsp
Tomato purée	0.5 tbsp	0.5 tbsp	0.5 tbsp	0.5 tbsp	0.5 tbsp	1 tbsp
Oregano, dried	0.5 tsp	0.5 tsp	0.5 tsp	0.5 tsp	0.5 tsp	1 tsp
Cheddar cheese	7 g	9 g	11 g	13 g	15 g	18 g

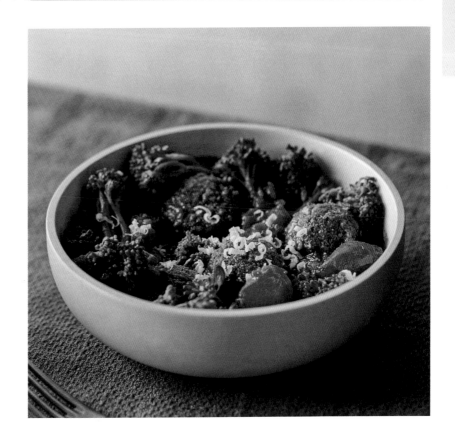

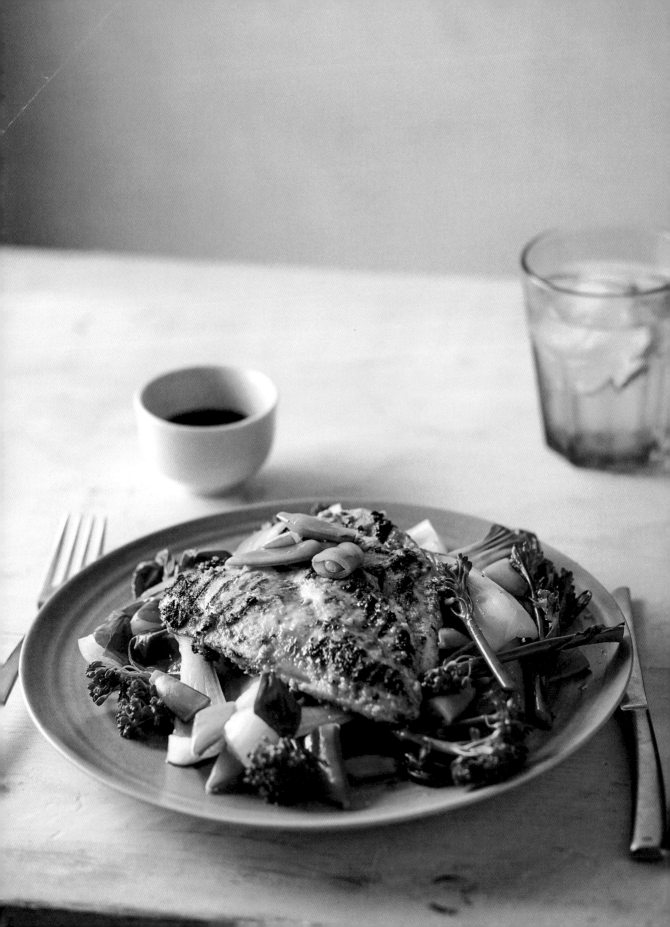

ASIAN PESTO CHICKEN WITH GREEN VEGETABLES

This meal is full of great flavours and is an awesome take on a classic pesto recipe with an Asian twist. This meal takes tasty healthy eating up a notch and beyond.

1. Butterfly the chicken breast, heat a skillet and fry until cooked through, flipping halfway, about 5 minutes each side.

2. Bring a pan of water to the boil and place the sugar snap peas, broccoli florets and pak choi in a steamer over the water to soften, about 4 minutes.

3. Make the pesto by blending the peanuts, honey, sweet chilli sauce, ginger, garlic, lemon juice, olive oil and coriander.

4. Serve the chicken with the pesto and green vegetables, seasoning with the soy sauce and some black pepper.

INGREDIENTS	1	2	3	4	5	6
Chicken breast	90 g	120 g	150 g	180 g	210 g	240 g
Sugar snap peas	60 g	80 g	100 g	120 g	140 g	160 g
Broccoli	42 g	56 g	70 g	84 g	98 g	112 g
Pak choi	42 g	56 g	70 g	84 g	98 g	112 g
Peanuts, roasted and salted	18 g	24 g	30 g	36 g	42 g	48 g
Honey	0.5 tsp	1 tsp	1 tsp	1 tsp	1.5 tsp	1.5 tsp
Sweet chilli sauce	0.5 tsp	1 tsp	1 tsp	1 tsp	1.5 tsp	1.5 tsp
Fresh ginger, crushed	0.5 tsp	1 tsp	1 tsp	1 tsp	1.5 tsp	1.5 tsp
Garlic, crushed	1 clove	1 clove	1 clove	1 clove	1 clove	2 cloves
Lemon juice	0.5 tbsp	1 tbsp	1 tbsp	1 tbsp	1.5 tbsp	1.5 tbsp
Olive oil	0.5 tsp	1 tsp	1 tsp	1 tsp	1.5 tsp	1.5 tsp
Coriander	1 handful	1 handful	1 handful	1 handful	1 handful	1 handful
Soy sauce	0.5 tsp	1 tsp	1 tsp	1 tsp	1.5 tsp	1.5 tsp

TUNA-STUFFED PEPPERS

Whoever came up with stuffing veg is a genius. This recipe is on that level. With some great ingredients packed into a sweet bell pepper, this dish is bursting with flavour.

1. Preheat the oven to 200°C/fan 180°C/gas mark 6.

2. Slice off the tops of the peppers, remove the seeds and white flesh inside and place on a baking tray. Cook 20 minutes, or until they are softened.

3. Meanwhile, fry the onion in the coconut oil on a medium heat for about 5 minutes until lightly browned, then add the garlic for a further 30 seconds.

4. Add the tuna steak and sweet potato to the pan and cover, flipping the tuna once halfway through, cooking for about 10 minutes until the it is cooked. Break the tuna apart and add the diced courgette. Remove from the heat once the courgette is cooked and add the mayonnaise and hot pepper sauce.

5. Remove the red pepper from the oven, fill with the tuna mix and top with a slice of mozzarella.

6. Return to the oven long enough to melt the mozzarella, about 5 minutes.

INGREDIENTS	1	2	3	4	5	6
Red pepper	1 pepper	1 pepper	1.5 peppers	2 peppers	2 peppers	2.5 peppers
Onion, diced	18 g	24 g	30 g	36 g	42 g	48 g
Coconut oil	0.5 tsp	1 tsp	1 tsp	1 tsp	1.5 tsp	1.5 tsp
Garlic, finely chopped	0.5 clove	0.5 clove	0.5 clove	1 clove	1 clove	1 clove
Tuna steak	96 g	128 g	160 g	192 g	224 g	256 g
Sweet potato, peeled and diced	18 g	24 g	30 g	36 g	42 g	48 g
Courgette, diced	36 g	48 g	60 g	72 g	84 g	96 g
Mayonnaise, reduced fat	24 g	32 g	40 g	48 g	56 g	64 g
Hot pepper sauce	1 tsp	1.5 tsp	2 tsp	2.5 tsp	3 tsp	3 tsp
Mozzarella, sliced	12 g	16 g	20 g	24 g	28 g	32 g

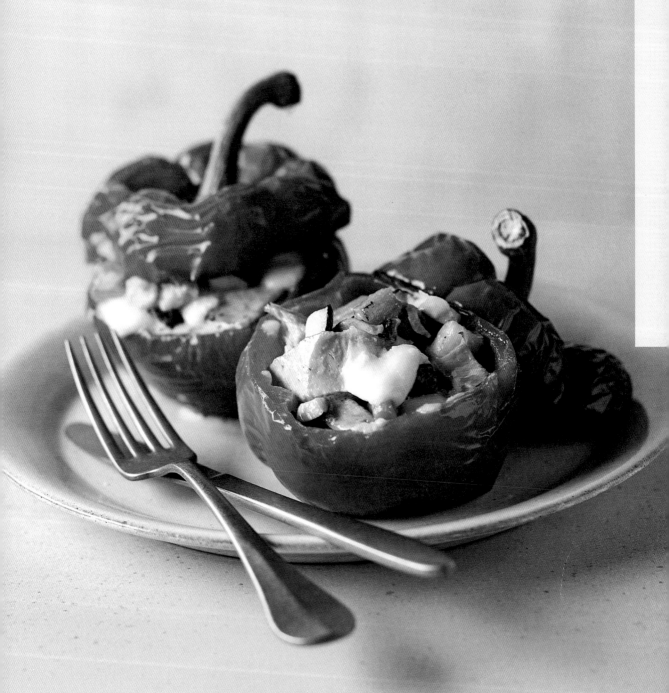

GINGER SESAME CHICKEN STIR-FRY WITH RICE NOODLES

This amazing Asian-style dish combines some tasty ingredients with numerous healthy additions, ginger being top of the pile.

1. Boil a pan of water and add the rice noodles. Cook until soft, about 7 minutes, then drain.

2. Meanwhile, heat the coconut oil in a pan then fry the strips of chicken with the grated ginger and sesame seeds, stirring frequently, for 3 minutes.

3. Add the carrot and courgette – cut into julienne strips – to the chicken with half the soy sauce. Stir-fry for a further 8 minutes.

4. Plate the noodles, pour over the remaining soy sauce and cover with the chicken stir-fry.

INGREDIENTS	1	2	3	4	5	6
Rice noodles	27 g	36 g	45 g	54 g	63 g	72 g
Coconut oil	0.5 tsp	0.5 tsp	1 tsp	1 tsp	1 tsp	1.5 tsp
Chicken breast, cut into strips	96 g	128 g	160 g	192 g	224 g	256 g
Fresh ginger, grated	1 cm	2 cm	2 cm	2 cm	3 cm	3 cm
Sesame seeds	1.5 tbsp	2 tbsp	2.5 tbsp	3 tbsp	3.5 tbsp	4 tbsp
Carrot, peeled and cut into thin strips	48 g	64 g	80 g	96 g	112 g	128 g
Courgette, cut into thin strips	48 g	64 g	80 g	96 g	112 g	128 g
Soy sauce	1 tsp	1.5 tsp	2 tsp	2.5 tsp	1 tbsp	1 tbsp

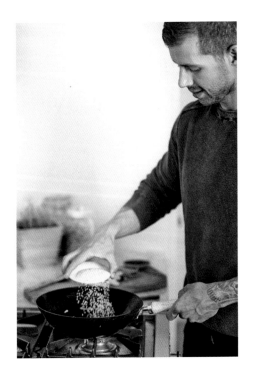
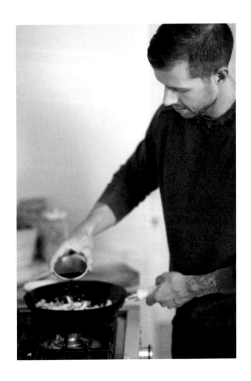
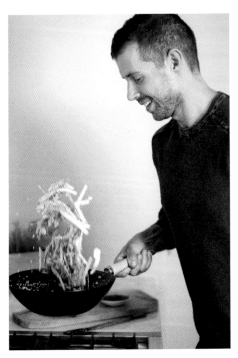
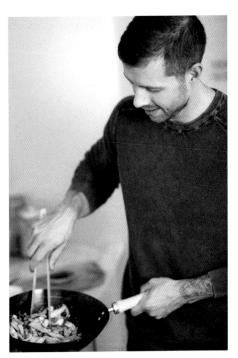

NEW YORK-STYLE OPEN PASTRAMI AND TURKEY SANDWICH

I've spent a fair amount of time in New York through work. And this is my go-to sandwich whenever I am out there. The addition of sliced turkey to this classic really adds a healthy boost. Having this great combination of flavours on a toasted slice of rye is a real treat.

1. Toast the bread and spread on the butter.

2. Mix the the mustard with the grated Parmesan and spread a thin layer on the bread.

3. Top with the gherkin slices then alternate layers of rocket, pastrami, turkey and the Parmesan-mustard mix to make the open sandwich. Enjoy.

note: slices of bread assume you are using a standard pre-sliced loaf of rye bread. If you are using dense 'pumpernickel' rye bread, use the weights given in brackets rather than slices.

INGREDIENTS	1	2	3	4	5	6
Rye bread	1 slice (30 g)	1 slice (40 g)	1½ slices (50 g)	1½ slices (60 g)	2 slices (70 g)	2 slices (80 g)
Butter	0.5 tsp	1 tsp	1 tsp	1 tsp	13 g	1.5 tsp
Parmesan cheese, grated	3 g	4 g	5 g	6 g	7 g	8 g
Wholegrain mustard	18 g	24 g	30 g	36 g	42 g	48 g
Rocket leaves	12 g	16 g	20 g	24 g	28 g	32 g
Pickled gherkin, finely sliced	0.5 small	1 small	1 small	1 small	1.5 small	1.5 small
Pastrami	55 g	70 g	90 g	110 g	125 g	145 g
Deli turkey	55 g	70 g	90 g	110 g	125 g	145 g

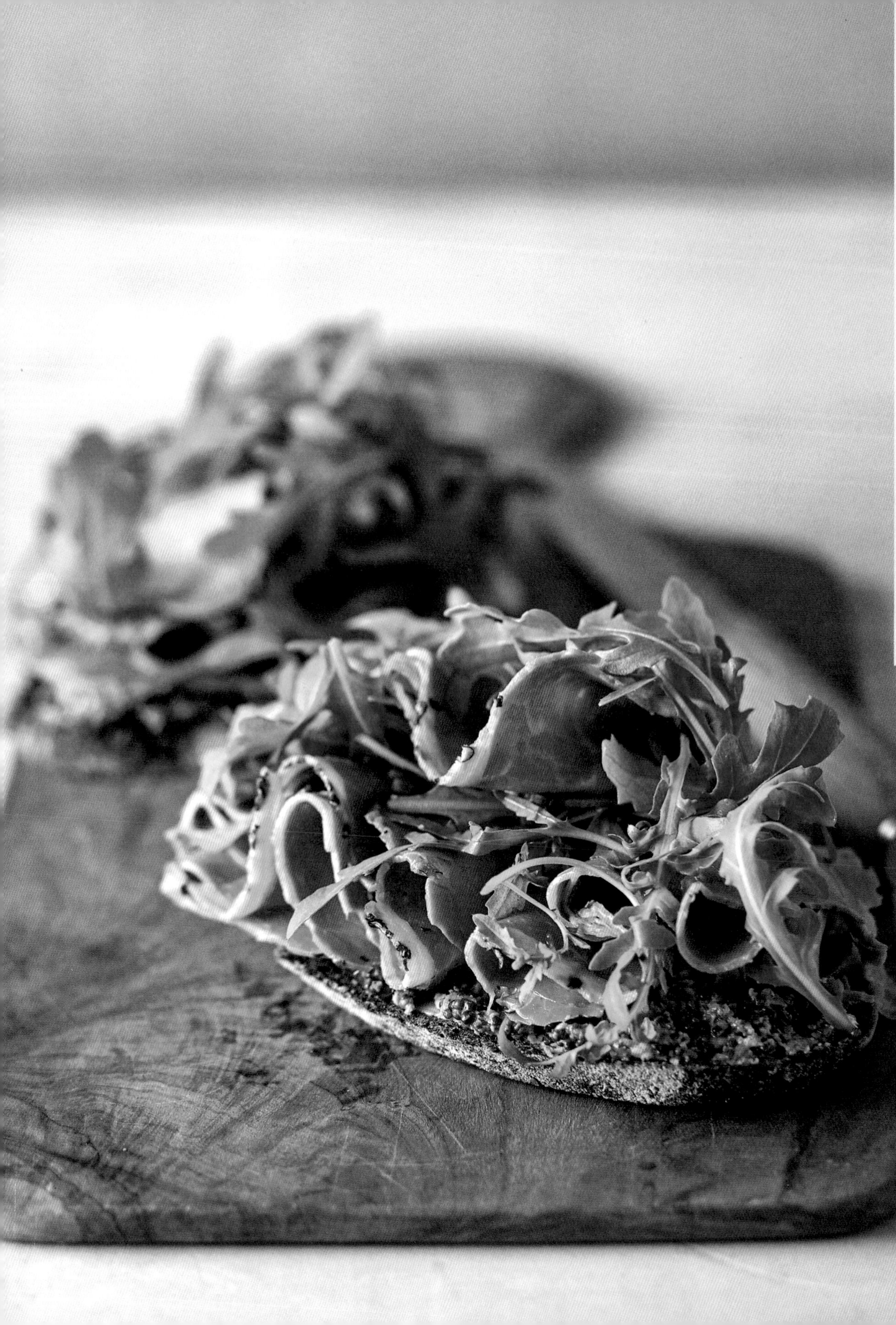

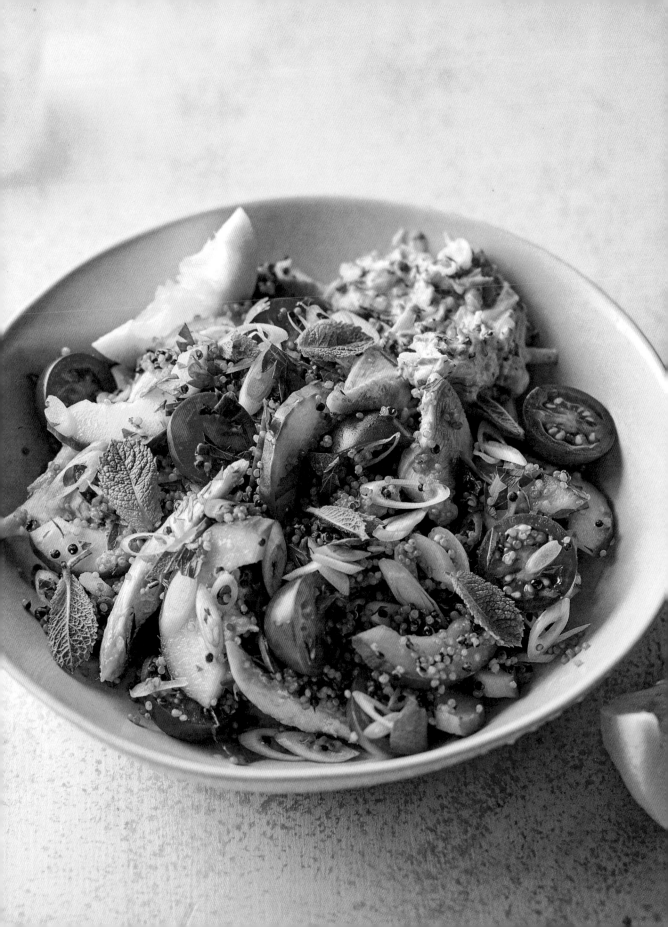

CHICKEN AND QUINOA TABBOULEH WITH TZATZIKI

This top Mediterranean meal takes fresh to another level, with a combination of ingredients that'll make you feel like you're on holiday in the sunshine.

1. Rinse the quinoa, cover with water and bring to the boil. Simmer for about 15 minutes, until cooked, then drain and cool.

2. Meanwhile, heat one-third of the oil in a pan, add the strips of chicken and fry until cooked, about 10 minutes.

3. To make the tzatziki: grate one-third of the cucumber and mix in a bowl with the Greek yogurt and half of the lemon juice, garlic and mint.

4. To make the tabbouleh: slice the remaining cucumber and mix with the cooked quinoa, tomatoes, spring onions, parsley, and the remainder of the lemon juice, garlic, mint and oil. Season the tabbouleh and serve with the chicken and tzatziki.

note: make sure you use Greek yogurt, as opposed to Greek-style yogurt

INGREDIENTS	1	2	3	4	5	6
Quinoa	24 g	32 g	40 g	48 g	56 g	64 g
Olive oil	2 tsp	2.5 tsp	3 tsp	3.5 tsp	4 tsp	5 tsp
Chicken breast, cut into strips	90 g	120 g	150 g	180 g	210 g	240 g
Cucumber	90 g	120 g	150 g	180 g	210 g	240 g
Greek yogurt, 0% fat	32 g	42 g	53 g	64 g	74 g	85 g
Lemon juice	1 tsp	1.5 tsp	2 tsp	2.5 tsp	3 tsp	3 tsp
Garlic	0.5 cloves	1 clove	1 clove	1 clove	1.5 cloves	1.5 cloves
Mint	1 handful	1 handful	1 handful	2 handfuls	2 handful	2 handfuls
Cherry tomatoes, halved	54 g	72 g	90 g	108 g	126 g	144 g
Spring onions, sliced	18 g	24 g	30 g	36 g	42 g	48 g
Parsley, chopped	2 tbsp	2 tbsp	3 tbsp	1 handful	1 handful	1 handful

SALMON PASTA SALAD WITH LEMON AND CAPERS

This is an awesome seafood salad with the saltiness coming from the capers and the salmon with lemon cutting through everything and ending on a fresh note.

1. Bring a large pan of water to the boil, add the pasta and simmer until al dente, about 11 minutes. Do not overcook as this will result in a mushy salad.

2. Heat the olive oil in a pan, add the slices of red pepper, cover and leave on a high heat for about 5 minutes to soften and char.

3. Push the pepper to one side, lower the heat to medium and add the salmon steak. Cover for about 10 minutes to cook through.

4. In a large bowl, mix the zest and juice of the lemon with the garlic, shallots and capers (if you prefer your shallots with less bite, soak in water for 10 minutes first, then drain).

5. Add the pepper and salmon, stir in the drained pasta and mix well, allowing the salmon to break apart.

6. Mix in the rocket leaves just before serving.

INGREDIENTS	1	2	3	4	5	6
Farfalle (bow-tie) pasta	18 g	24 g	30 g	36 g	42 g	48 g
Olive oil	0.5 tsp	0.5 tsp	0.5 tsp	0.5 tsp	0.5 tsp	1 tsp
Red pepper, sliced	48 g	64 g	80 g	96 g	112 g	128 g
Wild salmon steak	114 g	152 g	190 g	228 g	266 g	304 g
Lemon	0.5 lemon	0.5 lemon	0.5 lemon	0.5 lemon	0.5 lemon	1 lemon
Garlic, crushed	0.5 clove	1 clove	1 clove	1 clove	1.5 cloves	1.5 cloves
Shallots, finely chopped	18 g	24 g	30 g	36 g	42 g	48 g
Capers	1 tbsp	1.5 tbsp	2 tbsp	2.5 tbsp	3 tbsp	3 tbsp
Rocket leaves	24 g	32 g	40 g	48 g	56 g	64 g

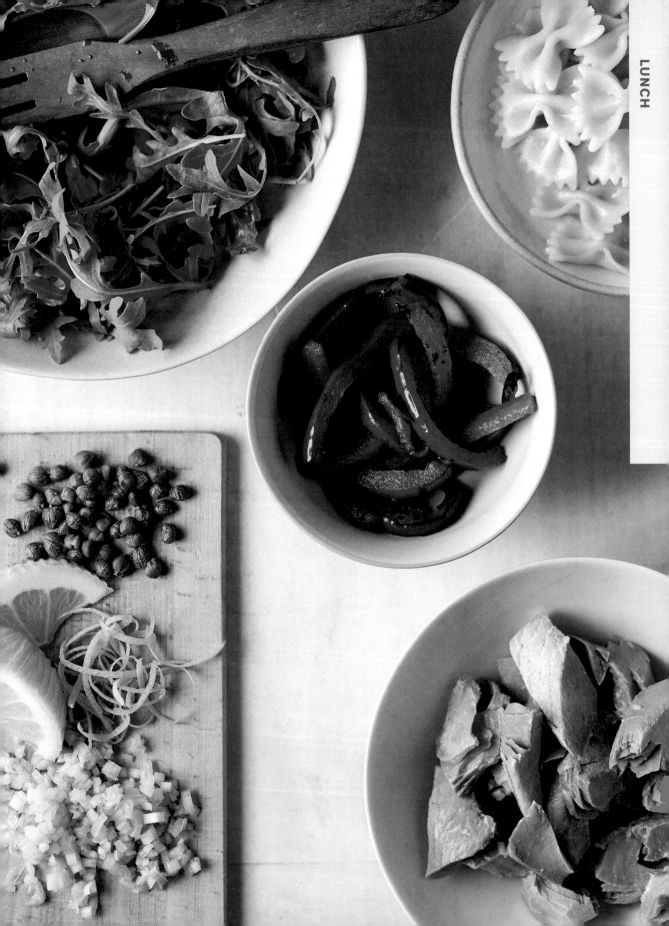

TEMPEH PAD THAI WITH SHIRATAKI NOODLES

I've eaten plenty of Pad Thais in my time, having spent many months in Thailand. This fresh-tasting and satisfying dish is one of my all-time favourites. Make sure you only use Skirtaki noodles - they are zero-carb noodles, so shouldn't be substitued for anything else.

1. Mix the fish sauce, the zest and juice of the lime, the sweet chilli sauce, garlic, chilli pepper and peanut butter in a bowl, then add the sliced tempeh and leave to soak up the flavours for at least 20 minutes.

2. Heat a frying pan on the hob, add the shallots and half the spring onions, and fry until golden-brown and fragrant.

3. Add the tempeh and its marinade to the pan, stir through and simmer for 5 minutes.

4. Meanwhile, bring another pan of water to the boil. Drain the noodles if pre-packed in liquid then add to pan and cook for 3 minutes. Drain, cover and set aside.

5. Push the tempeh mix to one side of frying pan, break in the egg and allow the white to set, then add the shirataki noodles and stir until all the ingredients are well combined.

6. Season and serve with fresh coriander and slices of the remaining spring onions.

INGREDIENTS	1	2	3	4	5	6
Fish sauce	0.5 tbsp	1 tbsp	1 tbsp	1 tbsp	1.5 tbsp	1.5 tbsp
Lime	0.5 limes	0.5 limes	0.5 limes	0.5 limes	0.5 limes	1 lime
Sweet chilli sauce	0.5 tbsp	1 tbsp	1 tbsp	1 tbsp	1.5 tbsp	1.5 tbsp
Garlic, crushed	1 clove	1 clove	1 clove	1 clove	1 clove	2 cloves

Red chilli pepper, finely chopped	9 g	12 g	15 g	18 g	21 g	24 g
Peanut butter	1 tsp	1.5 tsp	2 tsp	2.5 tsp	3 tsp	3 tsp
Tempeh, sliced	105 g	140 g	175 g	210 g	245 g	280 g
Shallots, finely chopped	24 g	32 g	40 g	48 g	56 g	64 g
Spring onions, sliced	18 g	24 g	30 g	36 g	42 g	48 g
Shirataki noodles	90 g	120 g	150 g	180 g	210 g	240 g
Eggs	1 small	1 small	1 medium	1 large	2 small	2 small
Fresh coriander	1 handful	1 handful	1 handful	1 handful	1 handful	1 handful

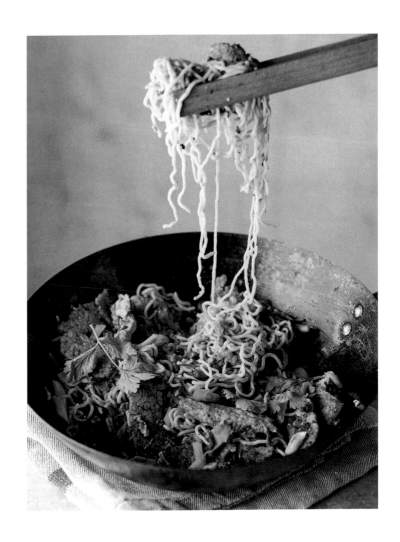

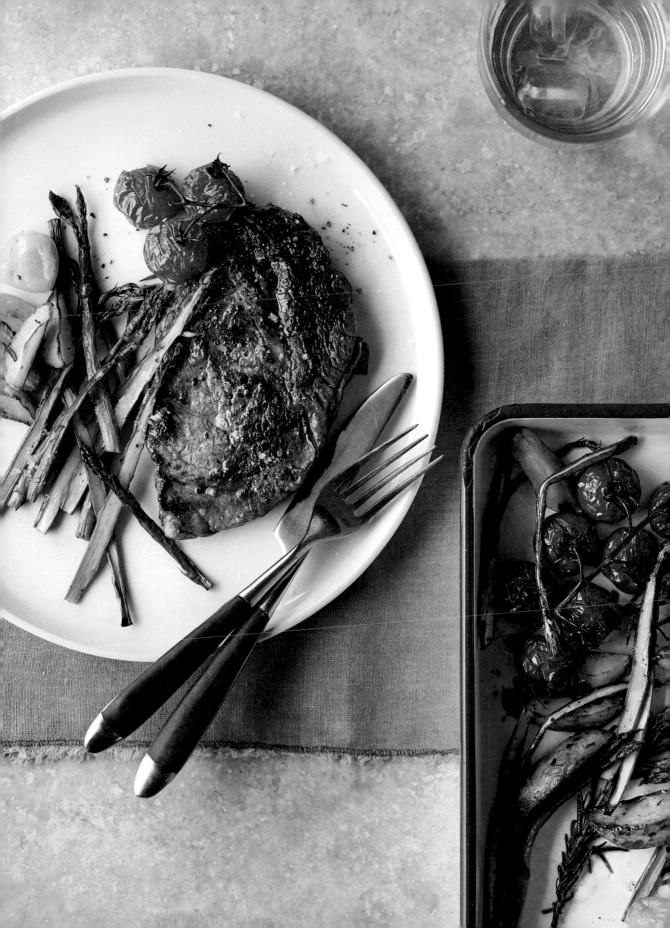

STEAK AND ROAST VEGETABLES

This is the kind of dish where you feel like you got a lot more than you bargained for. With the combination of steak and potatoes you can't go wrong in my book.

1. Preheat the oven to 180°C/fan 160°C/gas mark 4. Put the potatoes on a baking tray and sprinkle over half the coconut oil, rosemary and Worcestershire sauce. Roast in the oven for 20 minutes.

2. Add the asparagus and tomatoes to the baking tray, along with the remainder of the rosemary and Worcestershire sauce, and roast for a further 30 minutes.

3. Just before the vegetables are ready, fry the steak in the rest of the oil for a few minutes on each side, to preference.

INGREDIENTS	1	2	3	4	5	6
New potatoes, roughly chopped	60 g	80 g	100 g	120 g	140 g	160 g
Coconut oil	2 tsp	2.5 tsp	3 tsp	3.5 tsp	4.5 tsp	5 tsp
Rosemary, chopped	1 tbsp	1 tbsp	2 tbsp	2 tbsp	3 tbsp	3 tbsp
Worcestershire sauce	0.5 tsp	1 tsp	1 tsp	1 tsp	1.5 tsp	1.5 tsp
Asparagus	60 g	80 g	100 g	120 g	140 g	160 g
Cherry tomatoes	90 g	120 g	150 g	180 g	210 g	240 g
Beef steak	108 g	144 g	180 g	216 g	252 g	288 g

TUNA-STUFFED COURGETTE

These ingredients packed into the hollowed-out hull of a courgette become even more desirable when the dish is finished off with melted cheese sprinkled over the top.

1. Place the courgette on a baking tray and bake at 180°C/fan 160°C/gas mark 4 for 15 minutes.

2. Take the courgette out of the oven and carefully scoop out the centre.

3. Mix the soft courgette centre with the sweetcorn, yogurt and tuna, and put this mix back into the hollowed-out courgette shell.

4. Grate the cheese over the courgette and place back in the oven to bake for a further 20 minutes.

5. Serve alongside a salad of the cherry tomatoes with fresh parsley sprinkled on top.

note: these can be prepared the day before and heated up in the microwave, or enjoyed cold. Skyr can be substituted for any fat-free Greek yogurt.

INGREDIENTS	1	2	3	4	5	6
Courgette	96 g	128 g	160 g	192 g	224 g	256 g
Sweetcorn, tinned	72 g	96 g	120 g	144 g	168 g	192 g
Skyr natural yogurt	66 g	88 g	110 g	132 g	154 g	176 g
Tuna, tinned	42 g	56 g	70 g	84 g	98 g	112 g
Cheddar cheese, grated	31 g	42 g	52 g	62 g	73 g	83 g
Cherry tomatoes, halved	36 g	48 g	60 g	72 g	84 g	96 g
Parsley, finely chopped	1 handful	1 handful	1 handful	1 handful	1 handful	2 handful

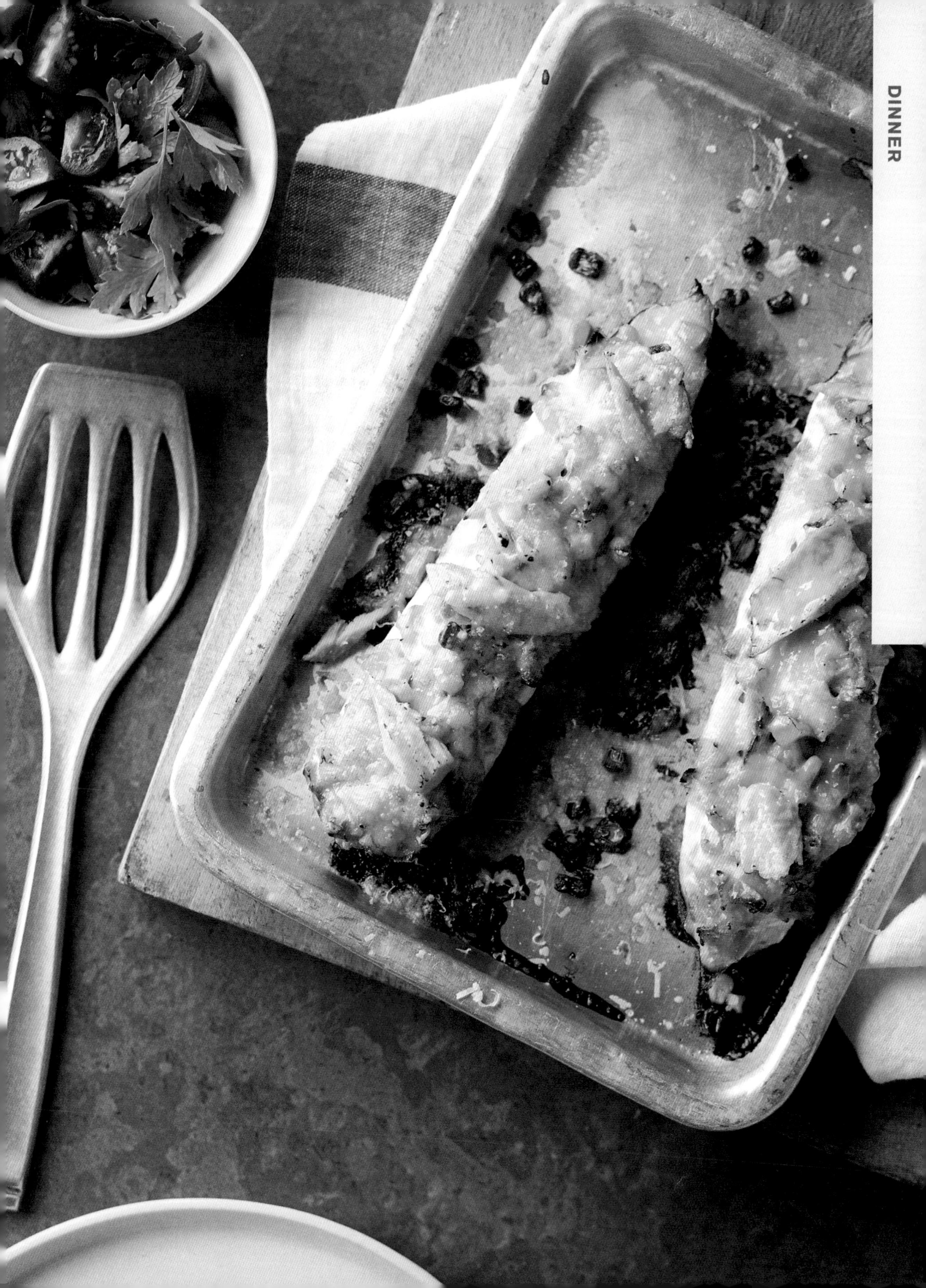

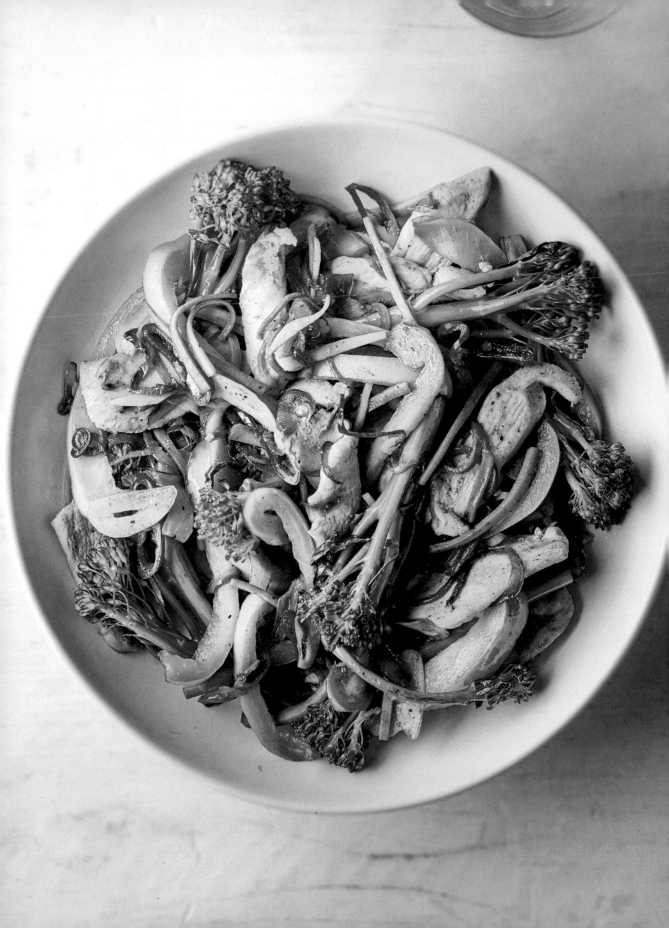

CHICKEN STIR-FRY

This is the perfect option if you fancy something with an Asian-style twist. It's hard to beat a stir-fry. With a mixture of freshness and heat combined with the flavours this recipe doesn't disappoint.

1. In a wok, heat the coconut oil, and add the sliced chicken. Cook for approximately 5 minutes on high heat.

2. Add the grated carrot, garlic, red onion, broccoli, orange pepper and chilli pepper. Fry for a further 5 minutes until the chicken is fully cooked.

3. Add the ginger and soy sauce and cook for a further 2 minutes.

4. Lastly, just before serving, add the sesame oil (this oil is normally tastier if not heated).

INGREDIENTS	1	2	3	4	5	6
Coconut oil	0.5 tbsp	0.5 tbsp	1 tbsp	1 tbsp	1.5 tbsp	1.5 tbsp
Chicken breast, sliced	99 g	132 g	165 g	198 g	231 g	264 g
Carrot, peeled and grated	24 g	32 g	40 g	48 g	56 g	64 g
Garlic, thinly sliced	0.5 clove	1 clove	1 clove	1 clove	1.5 cloves	1.5 cloves
Red onion, finely chopped	36 g	48 g	60 g	72 g	84 g	96 g
Broccoli, chopped	78 g	104 g	130 g	156 g	182 g	208 g
Orange pepper, chopped	96 g	128 g	160 g	192 g	224 g	256 g
Chilli pepper, finely chopped	12 g	16 g	20 g	24 g	28 g	32 g
Fresh ginger, finely chopped	1 cm	2 cm	2 cm	2 cm	3 cm	3 cm
Soy sauce	1 tbsp	1.5 tbsp	2 tbsp	2.5 tbsp	3 tbsp	3 tbsp
Sesame oil	1 tsp	1.5 tsp	2 tsp	2.5 tsp	3 tsp	3 tsp

BEEF STEW

This is a brilliant meal, especially if you own a slow cooker. The meat breaks apart so easily when cooked for this amount of time. It's also a perfect recipe for batch cooking.

1. Preheat the oven to 160°C/fan 140°C/gas mark 3. Thinly slice the garlic and roughly chop all the other veg into chunks.

2. Put all the vegetables, steak, tomato purée, sage and butter into an ovenproof casserole dish, and cover with boiling water.

3. Cover and bake for 3 hours. Alternatively, this can be cooked in a slow cooker on medium for 6–8 hours.

INGREDIENTS	1	2	3	4	5	6
Garlic	0.5 clove	1 clove	1 clove	1 clove	1.5 cloves	1.5 cloves
Green pepper	48 g	64 g	80 g	96 g	112 g	128 g
New potatoes	48 g	64 g	80 g	96 g	112 g	128 g
Carrot, peeled	36 g	48 g	60 g	72 g	84 g	96 g
Celery	36 g	48 g	60 g	72 g	84 g	96 g
Tomato purée	1 tbsp	1.5 tbsp	2 tbsp	2.5 tbsp	3 tbsp	3 tbsp
Onion	18 g	24 g	30 g	36 g	42 g	48 g
Stewing steak	114 g	152 g	190 g	228 g	266 g	304 g
Salted butter	1 tbsp	1.5 tbsp	1.5 tbsp	2 tbsp	2.5 tbsp	2.5 tbsp
Sage, chopped	1 handful	1 handful	1 handful	1 handful	1 handful	2 handful

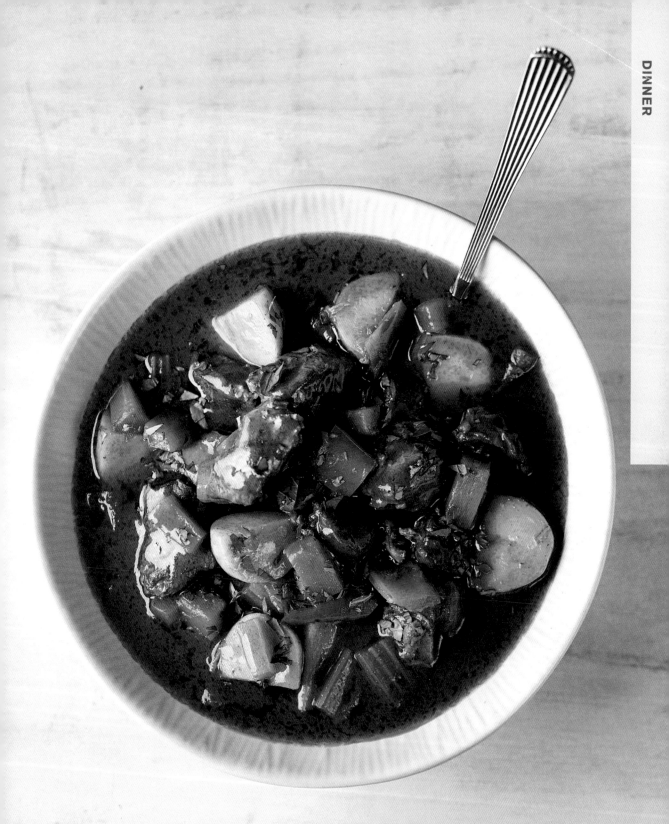

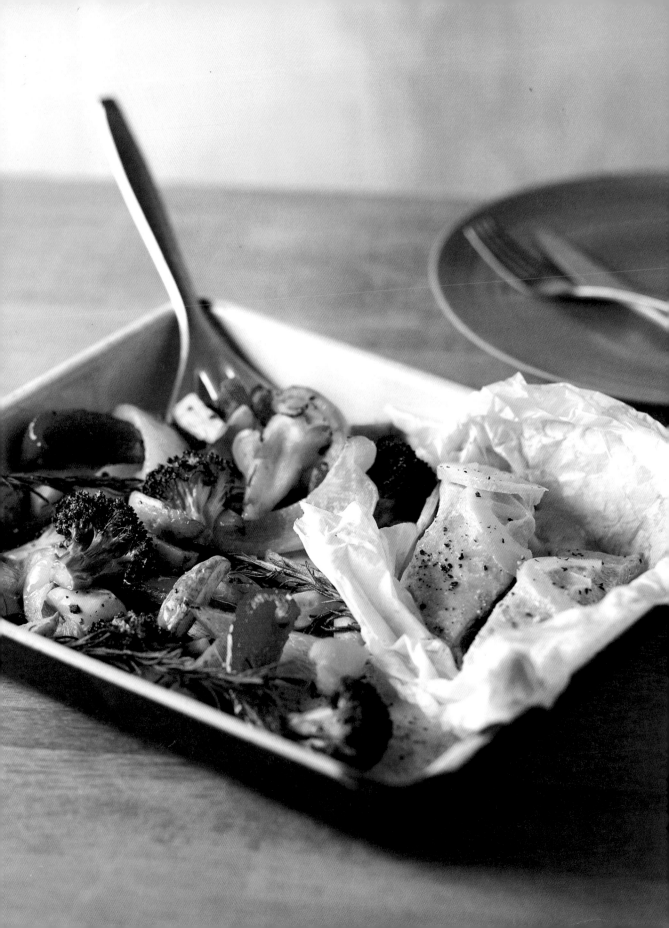

SALMON AND ROAST VEG

Cooking salmon in tin foil is an easy way to keep hold of the moisture and flavour of this delicious fish. This is a classy dish that requires minimal effort.

1. Preheat the oven to 180°C/fan 160°C/gas mark 4. Cut the veg into chunks, place on a baking tray with the rosemary and peppercorns and roast in the oven for 20 minutes.

2. Wrap the salmon steaks loosely in tin foil with the olive oil and slices of lemon. Bake with the veg for a further 20 minutes. Serve the salmon on top of the roasted veg.

note: ensure you use wild salmon for this recipe. Farmed salmon contains up to twice as much fat as wild salmon.

INGREDIENTS	1	2	3	4	5	6
New potatoes	51 g	68 g	85 g	102 g	119 g	136 g
Broccoli	48 g	64 g	80 g	96 g	112 g	128 g
Courgette	48 g	64 g	80 g	96 g	112 g	128 g
Red pepper	48 g	64 g	80 g	96 g	112 g	128 g
Yellow pepper	48 g	64 g	80 g	96 g	112 g	128 g
Rosemary	1 tbsp	1 tbsp	2 tbsp	2 tbsp	3 tbsp	3 tbsp
Peppercorns	0.5 tsp	1 tsp	1 tsp	1 tsp	1.5 tsp	1.5 tsp
Wild salmon steak	111 g	148 g	185 g	222 g	259 g	296 g
Olive oil	0.5 tsp	0.5 tsp	0.5 tsp	0.5 tsp	0.5 tsp	1 tsp
Lemon	0.5 lemon	0.5 lemon	0.5 lemon	0.5 lemon	0.5 lemon	1 lemon

PRAWN THAI GREEN CURRY

Another dish that takes me right back to my travels, this fragrant Thai green curry is packed with amazing flavours and always goes down a storm.

1. Thinly slice the aubergine, sweet potato and green beans and steam for 10 minutes.

2. Meanwhile, finely slice the shallots, red chilli and garlic and fry in a pan with the coconut oil and prawns for 3–5 minutes on a medium heat.

3. Halve the lemongrass lengthways then add it to the pan, along with the fish paste, lime leaves, coriander, fresh lime juice and coconut milk, and continue to cook for 5 minutes.

4. Add the steamed vgetables to the prawn mix and simmer for 10 minutes or until the aubergine is completely soft, then serve.

INGREDIENTS	1	2	3	4	5	6
Aubergine	48 g	64 g	80 g	96 g	112 g	128 g
Sweet potato, peeled	48 g	64 g	80 g	96 g	112 g	128 g
Green beans	36 g	48 g	60 g	72 g	84 g	96 g
Shallots	24 g	32 g	40 g	48 g	56 g	64 g
Red chilli	0.5	0.5	0.5	0.5	0.5	1
Garlic	0.5 clove	0.5 clove	0.5 clove	0.5 clove	0.5 clove	1 clove
Coconut oil	1 tsp	1.5 tsp	2 tsp	2.5 tsp	3 tsp	3 tsp
Prawns	156 g	208 g	260 g	312 g	364 g	416 g
Lemongrass	0.5 stalk	1 stalk	1 stalk	1 stalk	1.5 stalks	1.5 stalks
Fish paste	0.5 tbsp	1 tbsp	1 tbsp	1 tbsp	1.5 tbsp	1.5 tbsp
Kaffir lime leaves	2 leaves	2 leaves	3 leaves	4 leaves	4 leaves	5 leaves
Coriander, finely chopped	0.5 tbsp	1 tbsp	1 tbsp	1 tbsp	1.5 tbsp	1.5 tbsp
Lime juice	1 tsp	1.5 tsp	2 tsp	2.5 tsp	3 tsp	3 tsp
Light coconut milk	78 ml	104 ml	130 ml	156 ml	182 ml	208 ml
Basil	0.5 tbsp	1 tbsp	1 tbsp	1 tbsp	1.5 tbsp	1.5 tbsp

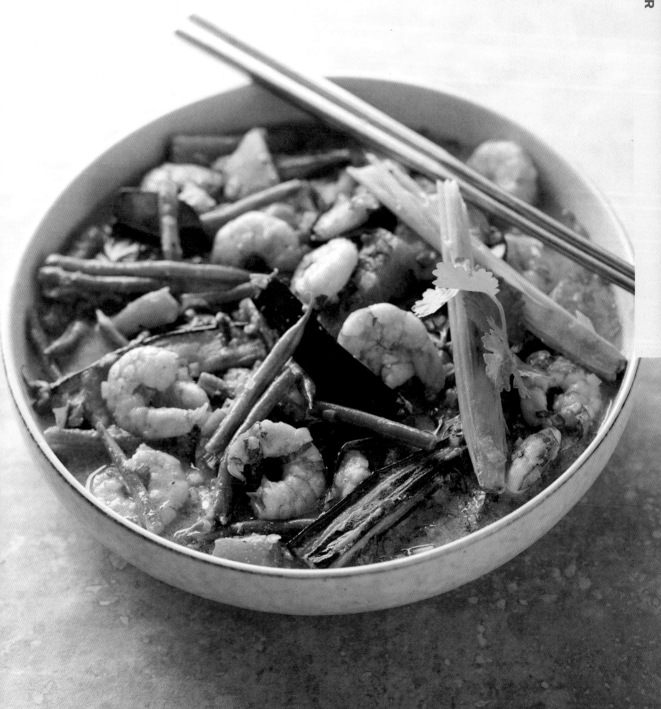

COD AMOK WITH SAUTÉED VEGETABLES

A traditional favourite in Cambodia, amok is an amazing-tasting dish that my mum has cooked many times for the family after her travels in that part of the world.

1. Preheat the oven to 180°C/fan 160°C/gas mark 4.

2. In a bowl, mix together the galangal (or ginger), garlic, coriander, turmeric and the rind and juice of half the lime. If your coconut oil is not liquid already, melt it and add half to the bowl, saving the rest for later.

3. Add the cod to the spices, stirring gently but being careful not to break apart the fish. Pour the contents of the bowl onto a large sheet of foil (or a large banana leaf if you have one).

4. Peel and cut the sweet potato into strips and lay alongside the fish. Fold over and seal the foil into a parcel to prevent moisture from escaping, then place on a baking tray and bake for 20 minutes for the smallest quantities, 30 for the largest.

5. For the last 5 minutes of the cooking time, place the flaked almonds on the baking tray alongside the fish to toast them lightly. Meanwhile, heat the remaining coconut oil in a pan and fry the broccoli for 3 minutes until softened.

6. Add the juice of the remaining lime and the kale to the broccoli and cook until wilted, about another 3 minutes.

7. Serve the fish and potato packet with the green vegetables topped with the toasted almonds, seasoned to taste.

INGREDIENTS	1	2	3	4	5	6
Galangal/fresh ginger, crushed	0.5 tbsp	1 tbsp	1 tbsp	1 tbsp	1.5 tbsp	1.5 tbsp
Garlic, crushed	1 clove	1 clove	1 clove	1 clove	1 clove	2 cloves
Coriander, chopped	1 handful	1 handful	1 handful	1 handful	1 handful	1 handful
Turmeric, ground	0.5 tsp	1 tsp	1 tsp	1 tsp	1.5 tsp	1.5 tsp
Lime	1 lime	1 lime	1 lime	1 lime	1 lime	2 limes
Coconut oil	1 tsp	1 tsp	1.5 tsp	2 tsp	2 tsp	2.5 tsp
Cod	123 g	164 g	205 g	246 g	287 g	328 g
Sweet potato	48 g	64 g	80 g	96 g	112 g	128 g
Flaked almonds	16 g	22 g	27 g	32 g	38 g	43 g
Broccoli, cut into florets	60 g	80 g	100 g	120 g	140 g	160 g
Kale	43 g	58 g	72 g	86 g	101 g	115 g

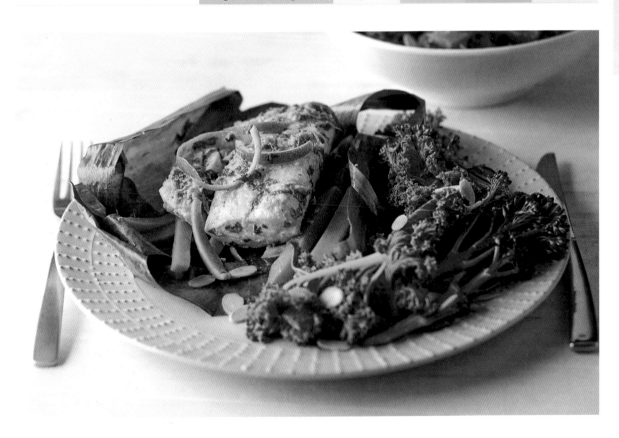

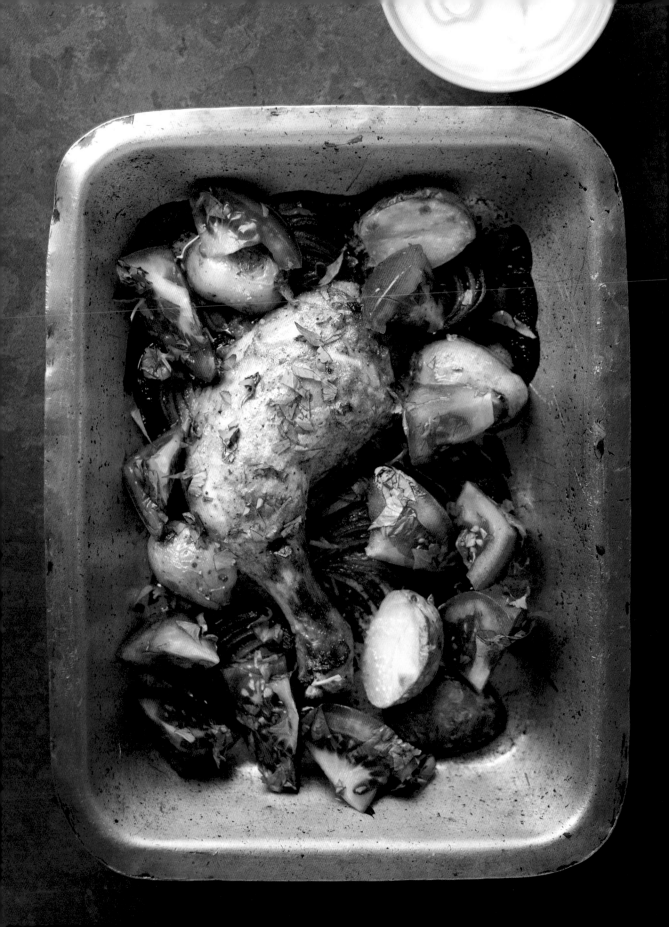

CURRIED CHICKEN AND NEW POTATO TRAY BAKE

The perfect meal for very little washing-up! Cooking in a single tray is a fantastic way to keep in all the flavours, letting them run through the other ingredients.

1. In a large bowl, mix together the garlic, ginger, curry spices and 2 tbsp of the Greek yogurt. Add the chicken thighs, coat well and leave to marinade for at least 1 hour.

2. Preheat the oven to 180°C/fan 160°C/gas mark 4. Place the chicken, sliced onion and new potatoes onto a baking tray, season well and bake for 40–60 minutes, until the potatoes are nicely golden and the chicken is cooked through.

3. Remove from the oven. Serve with the tomato dressed with the remaining Greek yogurt mixed with the lemon juice and coriander.

INGREDIENTS	1	2	3	4	5	6
Garlic, crushed	0.5 clove	1 clove	1 clove	1 clove	1.5 cloves	1.5 cloves
Ground ginger	0.5 tsp	1 tsp	1 tsp	1 tsp	1.5 tsp	1.5 tsp
Mixed curry spices	0.5 tsp	1 tsp	1 tsp	1 tsp	1.5 tsp	1.5 tsp
Greek yogurt, 0% fat	48 g	64 g	80 g	86 g	112 g	128 g
Chicken thigh, boneless with skin	120 g	160 g	200 g	140 g	280 g	320 g
Red onion, sliced	24 g	32 g	40 g	48 g	56 g	64 g
New potato, cut into chunks	60 g	80 g	100 g	120 g	140 g	160 g
Tomato, chopped	60 g	80 g	100 g	120 g	140 g	160 g
Coriander, finely chopped	1 handful	1 handful	1 handful	1 handful	1 handful	2 handfuls
Lemon juice	0.5 tbsp	1 tbsp	1 tbsp	1 tbsp	1.5 tbsp	1.5 tbsp

CHICKEN SKEWERS, CAULIFLOWER RICE AND GREEK SALAD

This is a great option with amazing flavours running through the chunks of marinated chicken, served alongside a tasty Greek salad and cauliflower rice.

1. In a large bowl, mix together the olive oil, vinegar, basil, coriander, lemon juice and garlic. Remove half the dressing and reserve for later.

2. Place the chicken pieces in the bowl, coat in the dressing and leave to marinade in the fridge for at least an hour.

3. Once marinated, skewer the chicken alternately with chunks of half the red pepper and place on a hot skillet to cook, turning a few times.

4. To make the cauliflower rice, chop the cauliflower into small pieces, then pulse in a food processor until it becomes the size of rice.

5. Put a pan over a medium heat, add half the red onion and fry until browned.

6. Then add the cauliflower rice and cover the pan. Cook until the rice is softened, about 5 minutes.

7. Meanwhile, make the salad by combining all the ingredients and dressing with the remaining oil mix from step 1. Serve with the chicken skewers and cauliflower rice and season to taste

INGREDIENTS	1	2	3	4	5	6
Olive oil	0.5 tsp	1 tsp	1 tsp	1 tsp	1.5 tsp	1.5 tsp
Red wine vinegar	0.5 tsp	1 tsp	1 tsp	1 tsp	1.5 tsp	1.5 tsp
Basil, chopped	6 leaves	8 leaves	10 leaves	12 leaves	14 leaves	16 leaves
Coriander, chopped	1 handful	1 handful	1 handful	1 handful	1 handful	2 handfuls
Lemon juice	0.5 tbsp	1 tbsp	1 tbsp	1 tbsp	1.5 tbsp	1.5 tbsp

Garlic, crushed	0.5 clove	1 clove	1 clove	1 clove	1.5 cloves	1.5 cloves
Chicken breast, cut into chunks	90 g	120 g	150 g	180 g	210 g	240 g
Red pepper, cut into chunks	96 g	128 g	160 g	192 g	224 g	256 g
Cauliflower	68 g	91 g	114 g	137 g	160 g	182 g
Red onion, finely chopped	36 g	48 g	60 g	72 g	84 g	96 g
Cucumber, sliced	33 g	44 g	55 g	66 g	77 g	88 g
Cherry tomatoes, halved	90 g	120 g	150 g	180 g	210 g	240 g
Feta cheese, cubed	21 g	28 g	35 g	42 g	49 g	56 g
Kalamata olives, stoned	21 g	28 g	35 g	42 g	49 g	56 g
Oregano, dried	0.5 tsp	1 tsp	1 tsp	1 tsp	1.5 tsp	1.5 tsp

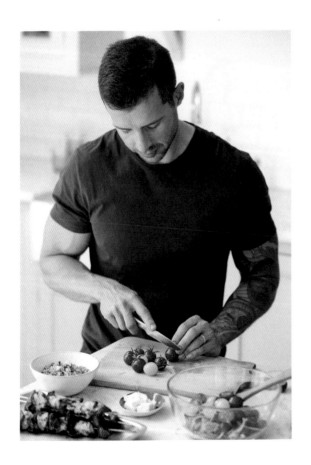

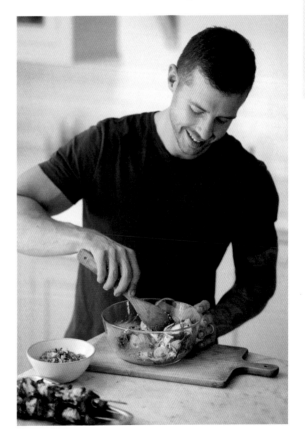

TUNA AND BEAN STIR-FRY

This fresh and juicy tuna can be served up in a matter of minutes with a heap of stir-fried veg.

1. Heat the coconut oil in a pan and add the onion, tuna, peas, spinach, green beans and mushrooms. Fry for 3 minutes.

2. Push the veg to one side of the pan and crack in the egg(s). Allow the white to set then stir the egg so it scrambles, but don't mix it into the veg.

3. Serve the veg topped with the egg, seasoned with pepper and soy

INGREDIENTS	1	2	3	4	5	6
Coconut oil	0.5 tbsp	1 tbsp	1 tbsp	1 tbsp	1.5 tbsp	1.5 tbsp
Onion, sliced	36 g	48 g	60 g	72 g	84 g	96 g
Tuna, tinned	66 g	88 g	110 g	132 g	154 g	176 g
Peas	48 g	64 g	80 g	96 g	112 g	128 g
Baby spinach	48 g	64 g	80 g	96 g	112 g	128 g
Green beans, halved	84 g	112 g	140 g	168 g	196 g	224 g
White mushroom, sliced	48 g	64 g	80 g	96 g	112 g	128 g
Eggs	1 medium	1 large	2 small	2 medium	3 small	3 small
Soy sauce	1 tbsp	1.5 tbsp	2 tbsp	2.5 tbsp	3 tbsp	3 tbsp

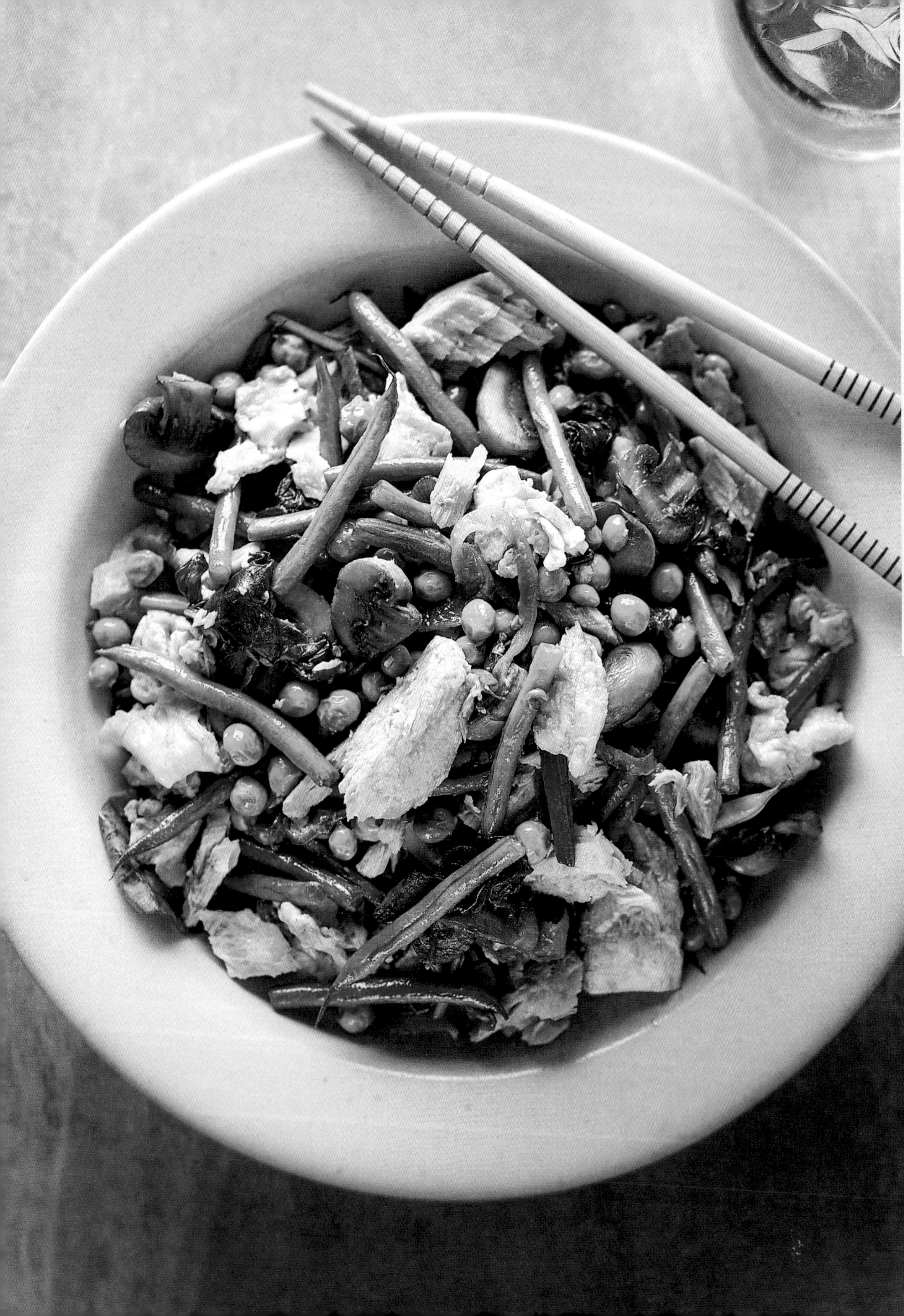

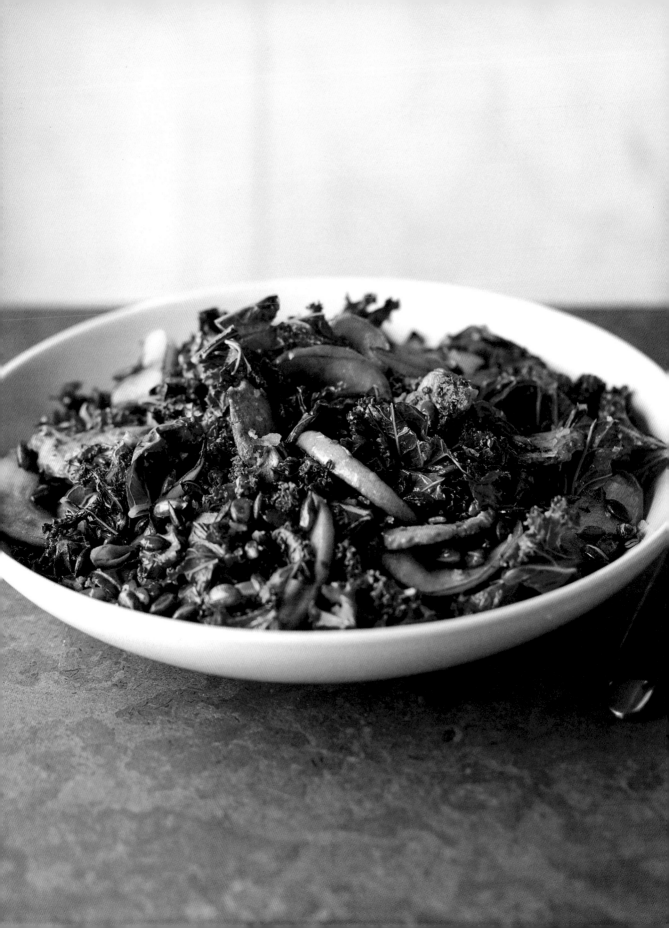

KALE AND PORK WITH SAUTÉED APPLE

There are many ingredients that work well together but pork and apple has a legendary status. Combined with the other ingredients, the pork is transformed into an awesome dinner.

1. In a small bowl, mix together the garlic, juice of half the lemon and two-thirds of the olive oil, adding a pinch of salt.

2. Cut the kale into ribbons and place in a large bowl with the zest of the lemon. Pour over the dressing and mix roughly.

3. Heat a pan with remainder of the oil, add the shallots and fry for a couple of minutes.

4. Add the sliced pork and fry for a couple of minutes on high.

5. Add the sliced apples and sauté until they soften and lose their bite, about 6–8 minutes on a medium heat. Mix the apples, shallots and pork into the bowl of kale.

6. Turn up the heat on the pan and add the pumpkin seeds. Toast on a high heat for 1–2 minutes, then add to the kale and apple.

7. Serve immediately or leave in the fridge to cool for later.

INGREDIENTS	1	2	3	4	5	6
Garlic, crushed	0.5 clove	1 clove	1 clove	1 clove	1.5 cloves	1.5 cloves
Olive oil	1 tbsp	1.5 tbsp	2 tbsp	2.5 tbsp	3 tbsp	3 tbsp
Curly kale	102 g	136 g	170 g	204 g	238 g	272 g
Lemon	1 lemon	1 lemon	1 lemon	1 lemon	2 lemons	2 lemons
Shallots, finely chopped	12 g	16 g	20 g	24 g	28 g	32 g
Apples, sliced	108 g	144 g	180 g	216 g	252 g	288 g
Pumpkin seeds	0.5 tbsp	1 tbsp	1 tbsp	1 tbsp	1.5 tbsp	1.5 tbsp
Pork, lean	108 g	144 g	180 g	216 g	252 g	288 g

FISH PIE WITH SWEET POTATO CRISP CRUST

When I'm lucky enough to eat out with my parents and fish pie is on the menu, my dad will be sure to order it. This dish goes a little further with the addition of sweet potato, making this recipe a family favourite.

1. Preheat the oven to 200°C/fan 180°C/gas mark 6.

2. Peel and roughly chop the sweet potato. Bring a pan of water to the boil, add the sweet potato to the pan and cook until very soft, about 20 minutes. Drain, season and mash.

3. While the potato is simmering, chop the cod into chunks and add to a hot, non-stick pan with the prawns, spinach and freshly squeezed lemon juice. Cook, stirring occasionally, until the spinach is fully wilted, then empty into a casserole dish. Stir in the crème fraîche.

4. Lay the sweet potato mash over the top of the fish. Grate over the Parmesan cheese and bake in the oven for 20–30 minutes, until top of the mash is lightly browned. Allow to cool for 10 minutes then serve.

INGREDIENTS	1	2	3	4	5	6
Sweet potato	54 g	72 g	90 g	108 g	126 g	144 g
Cod	90 g	120 g	150 g	180 g	210 g	240 g
Prawns	54 g	72 g	90 g	108 g	126 g	144 g
Spinach leaves	48 g	64 g	80 g	96 g	112 g	128 g
Lemon juice	0.5 tbsp	1 tbsp	1 tbsp	1 tbsp	1.5 tbsp	1.5 tbsp
Crème fraîche, full fat	2 tbsp	2.5 tbsp	3 tbsp	3.5 tbsp	4 tbsp	5 tbsp
Parmesan cheese	9 g	12 g	15 g	18 g	21 g	24 g

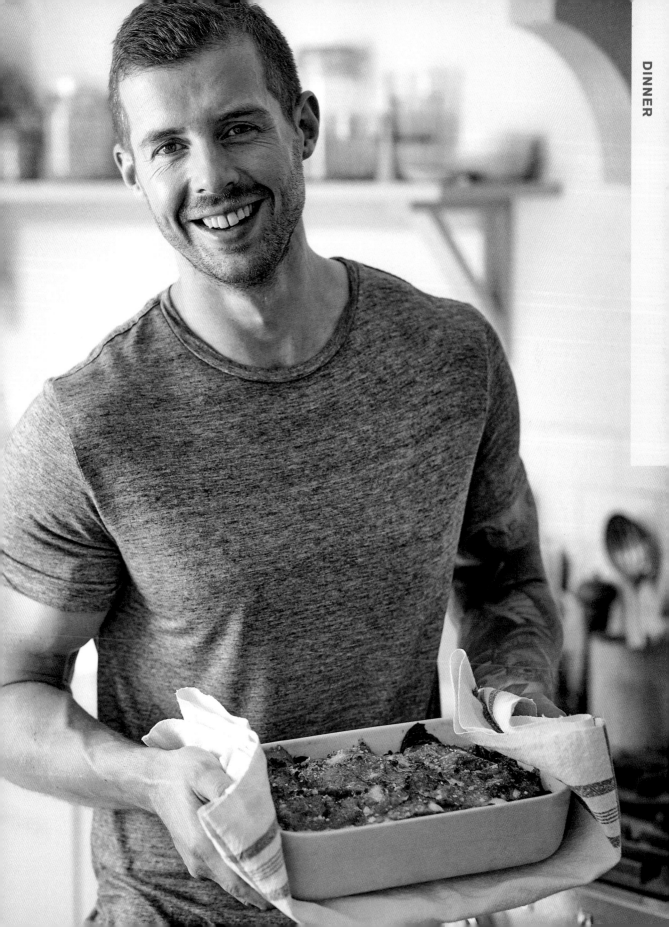

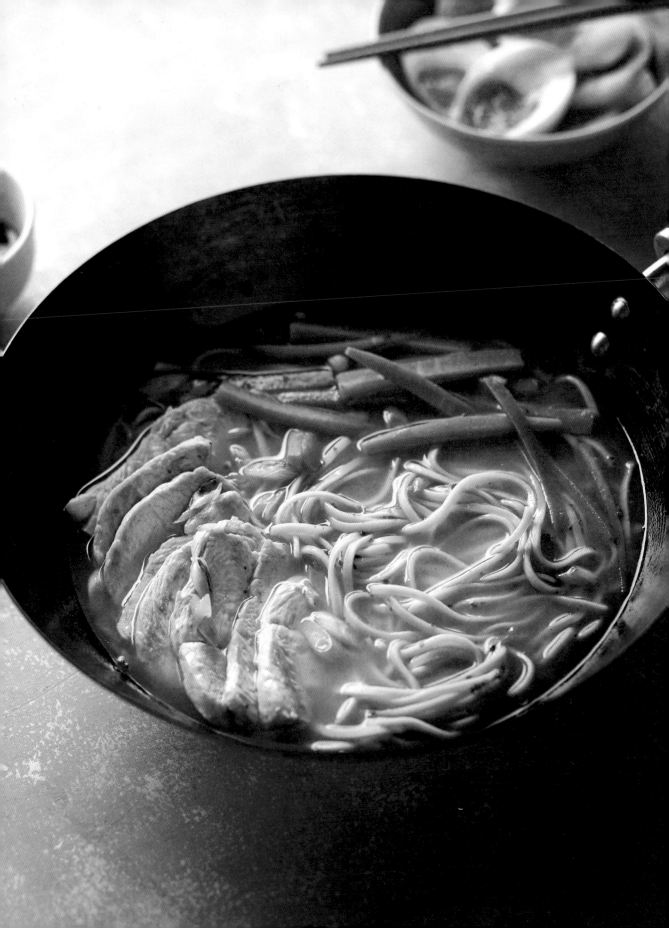

TURKEY AND EGG RAMEN

This Japanese option
is something a little
different that combines
a hearty bowl of ramen
noodles and turkey with a
fresh, satisfying broth.

1. Heat the sesame oil in a large pot, add the spring onions and fry until they are lightly browned, then add the turkey and carrot and fry for a further 5 minutes.

2. Boil the water, stir in the stock cube until it has dissolved and pour over the turkey. Add the kombu and simmer for 30 minutes.

3. Meanwhile, in a separate pan, bring some water to the boil, add the egg and boil for 6 minutes until hard boiled. Drain and pour over cold water to cool.

4. Add the noodles and soy sauce to the turkey broth and simmer for 2 minutes. Peel and halve the eggs, add to the ramen and serve.

INGREDIENTS	1	2	3	4	5	6
Sesame oil	1 tsp	1.5 tsp	2 tsp	2.5 tsp	3 tsp	3 tsp
Spring onion, chopped	18 g	24 g	30 g	36 g	42 g	48 g
Turkey, cut into chunks	72 g	96 g	120 g	144 g	168 g	192 g
Carrot, peeled and sliced	36 g	48 g	60 g	72 g	84 g	96 g
Water	180 ml	240 ml	300 ml	360 ml	420 ml	480 ml
Vegetable stock cube	0.5 cube	1 cube	1 cube	1 cube	1.5 cubes	1.5 cubes
Seaweed (kombu)	7 g	10 g	12 g	14 g	17 g	19 g
Eggs	1 large	2 small	2 medium	3 small	3 medium	3 large
Rice noodles	30 g	40 g	50 g	60 g	70 g	80 g
Soy sauce	0.5 tbsp	1 tbsp	1 tbsp	1 tbsp	1.5 tbsp	1.5 tbsp

TUNA AND ASPARAGUS WITH KIDNEY BEANS

This is a great meal that feels almost like a light curry, with some real freshness running through the flavours.

1. Grate the lemon zest, mix with the salt, pepper and ginger, and rub it into the tuna steak. Heat the coconut oil in a pan and add the tuna, along with the asparagus and sliced pepper, and cook for a few minutes each side until the vegetables have softened and the tuna is cooked to taste.

2. Meanwhile, mix the drained kidney beans and coconut milk in another pan and heat through.

3. Serve the kidney beans and tuna garnished with the chives and sprinkled with the juice of the lemon.

INGREDIENTS	1	2	3	4	5	6
Lemon	0.5 lemon	0.5 lemon	0.5 lemon	0.5 lemon	0.5 lemon	1 lemon
Salt	0.5 tsp	0.5 tsp	0.5 tsp	0.5 tsp	0.5 tsp	1 tsp
Black pepper	0.5 tsp	0.5 tsp	0.5 tsp	0.5 tsp	0.5 tsp	1 tsp
Ground ginger	0.5 tsp	0.5 tsp	0.5 tsp	0.5 tsp	0.5 tsp	1 tsp
Tuna steak	90 g	120 g	150 g	180 g	210 g	240 g
Coconut oil	1 tsp	1.5 tsp	2 tsp	2.5 tsp	3 tsp	3 tsp
Asparagus	90 g	120 g	150 g	180 g	210 g	240 g
Red pepper, sliced	60 g	80 g	100 g	120 g	140 g	160 g
Kidney beans, tinned	60 g	80 g	100 g	120 g	140 g	160 g
Coconut milk, tinned	36 g	48 g	60 g	72 g	84 g	96 g
Chives, finely chopped	0.5 tbsp	1 tbsp	1 tbsp	1 tbsp	1.5 tbsp	1.5 tbsp

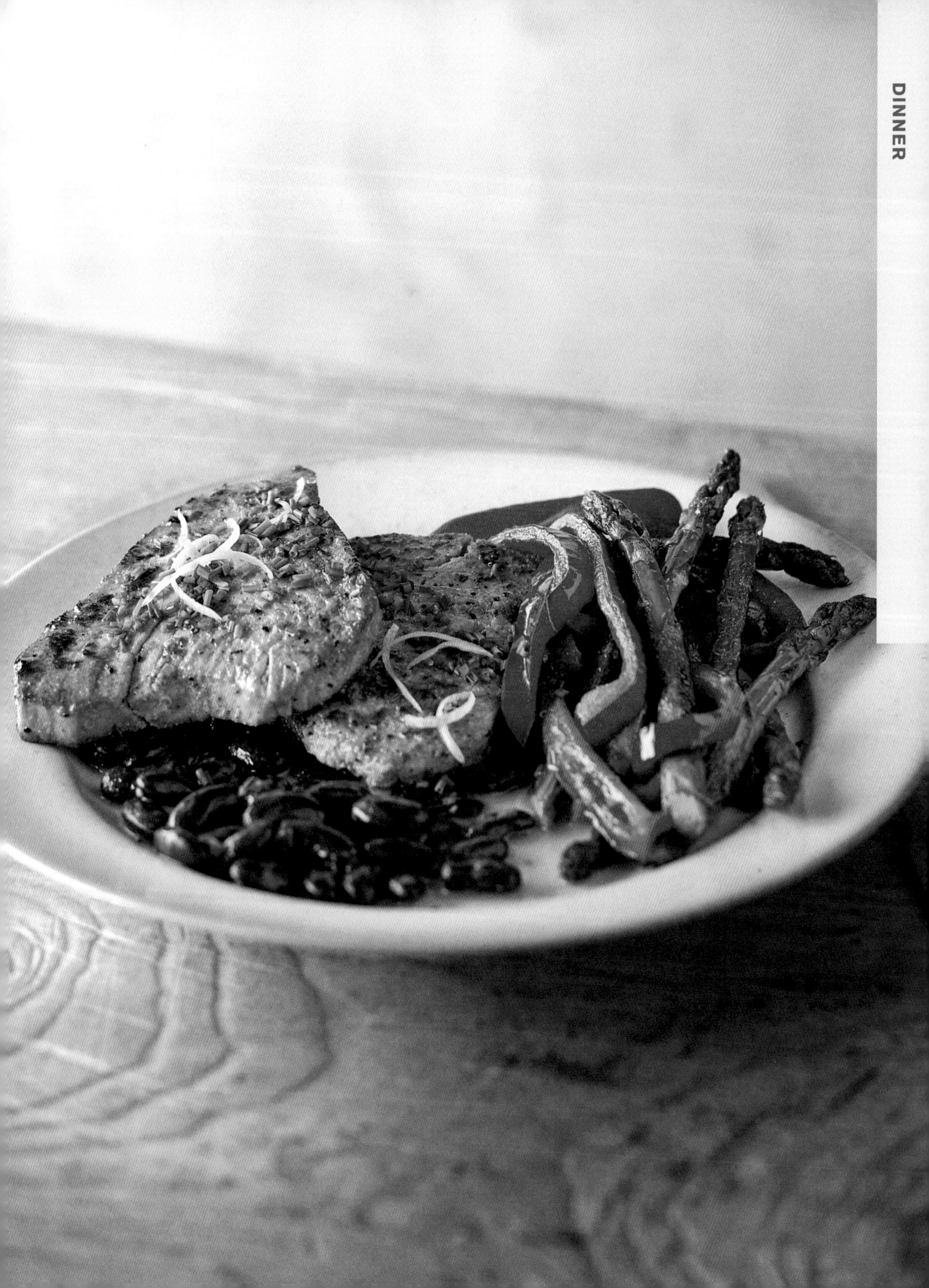

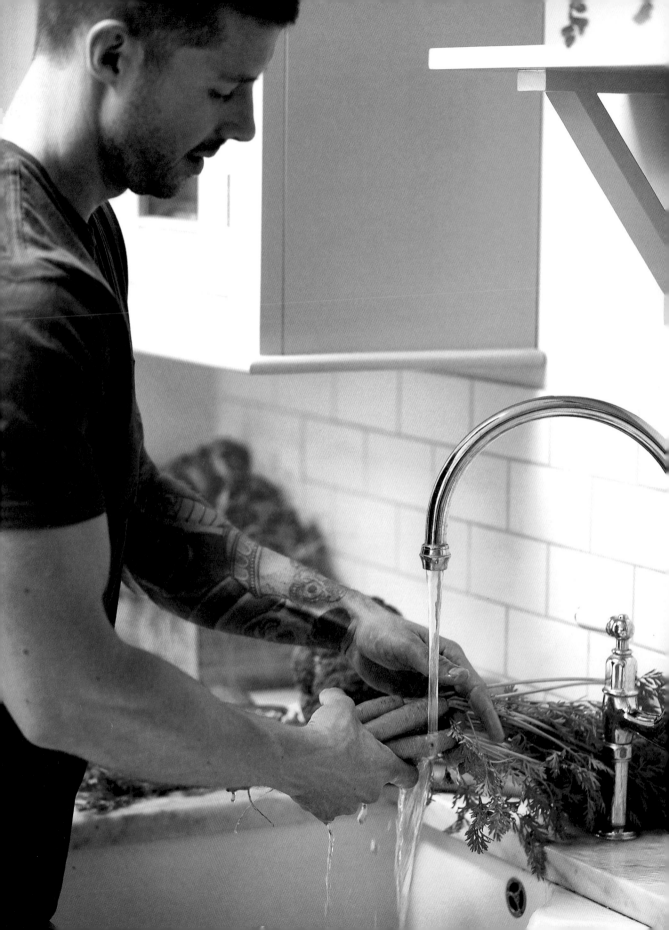

BREADED TUNA STEAK WITH GREENS

This is a great option if you fancy something with a little texture. Having the breaded crust really gives the tuna a different twist.

1. Combine the breadcrumbs, garlic, parsley and olive oil in a bowl, and mix together. Slowly squeeze lemon juice over the mixture until it forms a paste. This will be about half the juice from the lemon.

2. Season the tuna steak to taste with a pinch of salt, then cover both sides of the steak in the breadcrumb mixture, pressing down to ensure an even coating.

3. Cook in a hot pan for about 3 minutes each side.

4. Meanwhile, heat the coconut oil in another pan, add the spinach and broccoli and cover for about 5 minutes to cook the broccoli and wilt the spinach.

5. Serve the tuna and greens with a drizzle of the remaining lemon juice, adding pepper to taste.

INGREDIENTS	1	2	3	4	5	6
Breadcrumbs	18 g	24 g	30 g	36 g	42 g	48 g
Garlic, finely chopped	0.5 clove	0.5 clove	0.5 clove	0.5 clove	0.5 clove	1 clove
Parsley, finely chopped	2 tbsp	2 tbsp	3 tbsp	1 handful	1 handful	1 handful
Extra virgin olive oil	0.5 tbsp	1 tbsp	1 tbsp	1 tbsp	1.5 tbsp	1.5 tbsp
Lemon	0.5 lemons	0.5 lemons	0.5 lemons	0.5 lemons	0.5 lemons	1 lemon
Tuna steak	102 g	136 g	170 g	204 g	238 g	272 g
Coconut oil	0.5 tbsp	0.5 tbsp	0.5 tbsp	0.5 tbsp	0.5 tbsp	1 tbsp
Baby spinach	60 g	80 g	100 g	120 g	140 g	160 g
Broccoli, cut into florets	30 g	40 g	50 g	60 g	70 g	80 g

There are two types of snack on the following pages, high-carb snacks and low-carb snacks – flick back to page 37 to jog your memory as to which you can have on your plan. The recipes might seem quite large. This isn't an accident! The reason for this is to allow for greater variation in macros on resistance and non-resistance days, utilising a carb-cycling approach. Feel free to split the snacks into two portions to eat throughout the day if you'd prefer.

HIGH-CARB SNACKS

Eat these on resistance training days only (if your waist measurement is below the cut-off). They provide the perfect blend of carbs and protein for recovery from resistance training.

The high-carb snacks are set at 40 per cent calories from carbs, 40 per cent calories from protein and 20 per cent calories from fats. The additional carbs here are for recovery and energy and can be included on these days to fuel workouts and replenish muscle glycogen.

LOW-CARB SNACKS

If your waist measurement is above the cut-off these are your snacks each day of the week. If your measurement is below the cut-off, eat these on the days you're not doing resistance training.

They work in a very similar way to the main meals, with the majority of the energy coming from fat and protein. The macros have been balanced in this way to provide energy with a low impact on your blood sugar levels.

note: Many of these recipes use whey protein. You can use flavoured or unflavoured whey protein, and you can find good quality whey on my website.

APPLE CINNAMON BALLS

Apple and cinnamon is a flavour combination that works really well in this recipe. All of this with no cooking time at all – unless you consider the melting of the chocolate to be cooking!

1. Blend the oats to a fine powder and mix with the protein powder, apple sauce and cinnamon. Roll the mixture into balls.

2. Melt the chocolate and drizzle over the protein balls. Allow to set then enjoy.

INGREDIENTS	A	B
Oats	34 g	45 g
Whey protein	28 g	37 g
Apple sauce	1 tbsp	1 tbsp
Ground cinnamon	1 tsp	1 tsp
Dark chocolate (70–85% cocoa)	10 g	13 g

PROTEIN BIRCHER BOWLS

This is a great-tasting snack that is ideal for prepping ahead of time. You can even leave it overnight; it is simply and easily put together while cooking dinner in the evening to be ready the next morning.

note: Skyr can be substituted for low-sugar, fat-free Greek yogurt.

1. Mix the oats with the almond milk and leave to soak in the fridge for at least 2 hours, or overnight.

2. Mix the yogurt, whey protein, apple and cinnamon with the soaked oats. Sprinkle with the crushed pistachios to serve.

INGREDIENTS	A	B
Oat flakes, rolled	30 g	40 g
Almond milk, unsweetened	60 ml	80 ml
Skyr natural yogurt	53 g	70 g
Whey protein	20 g	27 g
Apple, grated	40 g	53 g
Ground cinnamon	1 tsp	1 tsp
Pistachio kernels, crushed	8 nuts	11 nuts

CHOCOLATE BANANA PROTEIN SHAKE

A simple shake with a lot to offer, this classic combination of chocolate and banana doesn't disappoint.

1. Blend everything together and drink.

INGREDIENTS	A	B
Oat milk, unsweetened	113 g	150 g
Banana	60 g	80 g
Apple sauce	45 g	60 g
Whey protein	30 g	40 g
Cocoa powder	1 tbsp	1 tbsp
Ground cinnamon	1 tsp	1 tsp
Chia seeds	1 tsp	1 tsp

BANANA AND BERRY SMOOTHIE

This is another simple shake with more of a fruity tone running through it. It is a great snack that can be quickly made at the start of a busy day. Make sure you use proper Greek yogurt instead of Greek style yogurt – the latter often contains much less protein, and you need around 9g per 100g for this.

1. Blend everything together and drink.

INGREDIENTS	A	B
Coconut water	113 ml	150 ml
Bananas	105 g	140 g
Greek yogurt, 0% fat	56 g	75 g
Blackberries	6 blackberries	8 blackberries
Raspberries	6 raspberries	8 raspberries
Whey protein	26 g	35 g

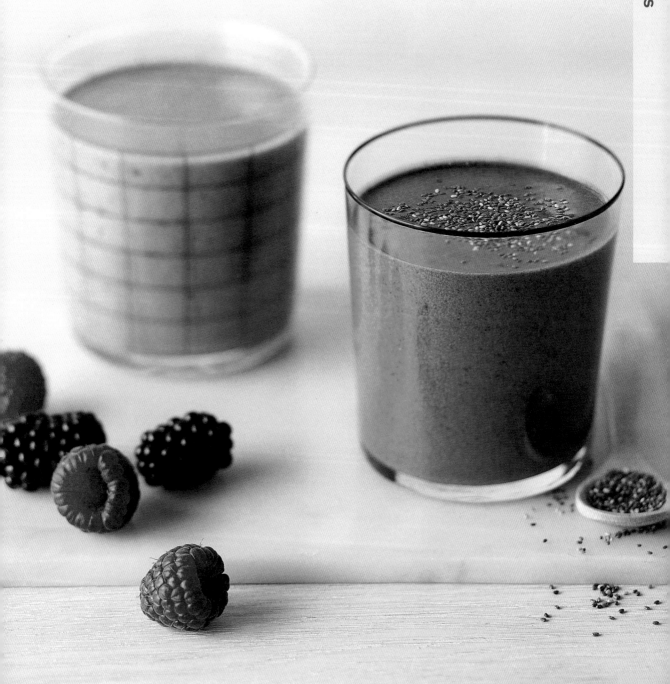

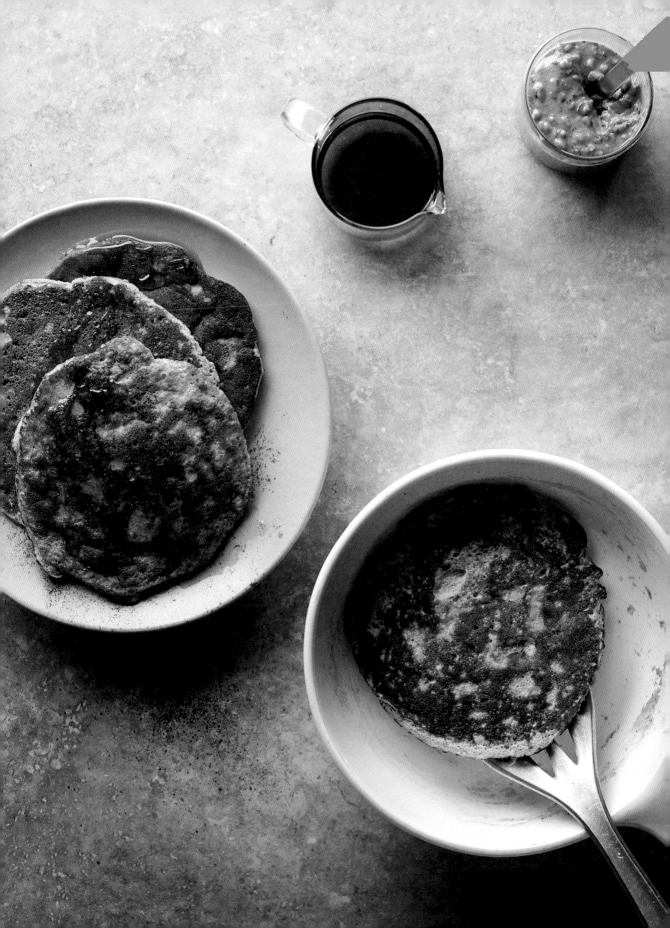

BANANA PANCAKES

You may feel like you're overindulging, but no – you're not when it's within your macros! With this recipe, you can have pancakes for breakfast and as a snack on the same day.

1. Mash the banana in a bowl with the back of a fork.

2. Add the protein powder, egg and egg white, baking powder and cinnamon and mash together. A few banana lumps left is fine.

3. Heat a non-stick frying pan on high, add the banana mix to the pan, and cook for a few minutes, flipping the pancakes halfway through when bubbles form across the surface.

4. Serve with maple syrup and peanut butter.

INGREDIENTS	A	B
Banana	94 g	125 g
Whey protein	23 g	30 g
Egg	1 small	1 medium
Egg white	1 small	1 medium
Baking powder	1 tsp	1 tsp
Ground cinnamon	1 tsp	1 tsp
Maple syrup	1 tbsp	1 tbsp
Peanut butter	1 tsp	1 tsp

BLUEBERRY OAT MUFFINS

These blueberry muffins are the best! Perfect for batch cooking, they are worth making over and over again. They almost have too much to offer. Make sure you use proper Greek yogurt instead of Greek *style* yogurt – the latter often contains much less protein, and you need around 9g per 100g for this.

1. Preheat the oven to 180°C/fan 160°C/gas mark 4 and line a muffin tray with cases. If you're making a 300-calorie snack then use the mixture to make eight muffins and eat 2 as one portion, and if you're making a 400-calorie snack make 9 muffins and have 3 for one portion.

2. Put one-third of the oats in a high-speed blender, and blend to a fine powder.

3. In a large bowl, mix together this oat flour, the remaining oats, protein powder, baking powder, cinnamon, bicarbonate of soda and salt.

4. In a separate bowl, whisk the egg and mix in the yogurt, maple syrup, almond milk (saving 1 teaspoon for later) and vanilla essence.

5. Combine the wet and dry ingredients, and mix in the blueberries. Divide the mixture evenly into the muffin cases.

6. Bake for 20–25 minutes, until a cake tester or toothpick comes out clean.

7. Melt the chocolate, add the saved teaspoon of almond milk, and drizzle over the muffins.

8. If making A snacks, make eight muffins and eat two muffins per snack; if making B snacks, make nine muffins and eat three muffins per snack.

INGREDIENTS

Oat flakes, rolled	100 g
Whey protein	85 g

Baking powder	2 tsp
Ground cinnamon	1 tsp
Bicarbonate of soda	0.5 tsp
Salt	1 pinch
Eggs	1 medium
Greek yogurt, 0% fat	225 g
Maple syrup	20 g
Almond milk, unsweetened	60 ml
Vanilla essence	2 tsp
Blueberries	140 g
Dark chocolate (70–85% cocoa)	30 g

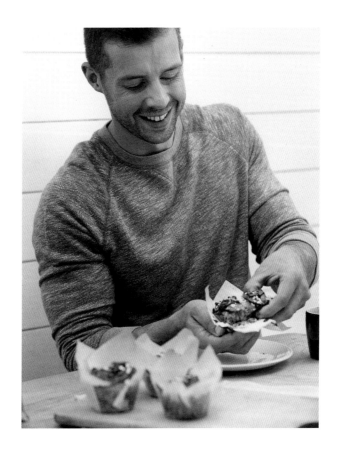

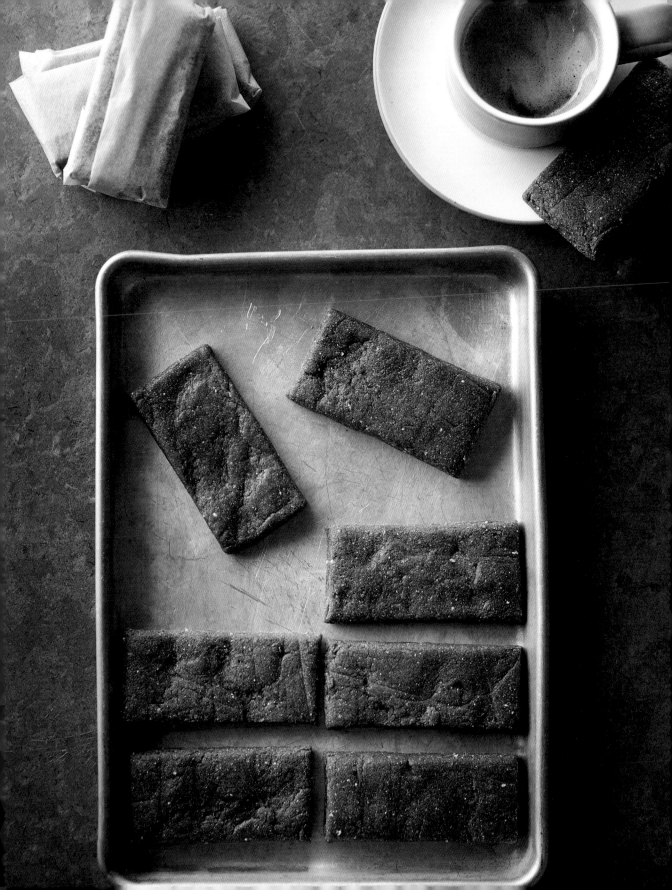

CHOCOLATE COFFEE PROTEIN BARS

Bite-sized protein bars are my idea of great convenience. Especially when they include one of my favourite flavours . . . coffee! You'll be sure to love this ingenious take on a standard protein bar.

1. Mix the protein powder, oat flour, coconut flour and cocoa powder in a bowl.

2. In a separate bowl, heat the peanut butter in the microwave until it is soft, then mix in the maple syrup and espresso shot.

3. Combine the wet and dry ingredients and press the mixture into a small baking tray. Cool for at least 30 minutes in the fridge.

4. If making A snacks, divide the mixture into four bars and have one a day. If making B snacks, divide into three bars and have one a day.

INGREDIENTS

Whey protein	110 g
Oat flour	100 g
Coconut flour	40 g
Cocoa powder	1 tbsp
Peanut butter, smooth	1 tbsp
Maple syrup	50 ml
Shot of brewed espresso	30 ml

BANANA CINNAMON YOGURT POT

With only three ingredients, this protein-packed snack is so simple – but it doesn't disappoint on flavour.

1. Slice the banana and mix it into the yogurt with the cinnamon.

note: do not use Greek *style* yogurt instead of Greek yogurt – it often contains much less protein. Make sure the yogurt you use is at least 9g protein per 100g.

INGREDIENTS	A	B
Banana	105 g	140 g
Greek yogurt, 0% fat	263 g	350 g
Ground cinnamon	1.5 tsp	2 tsp

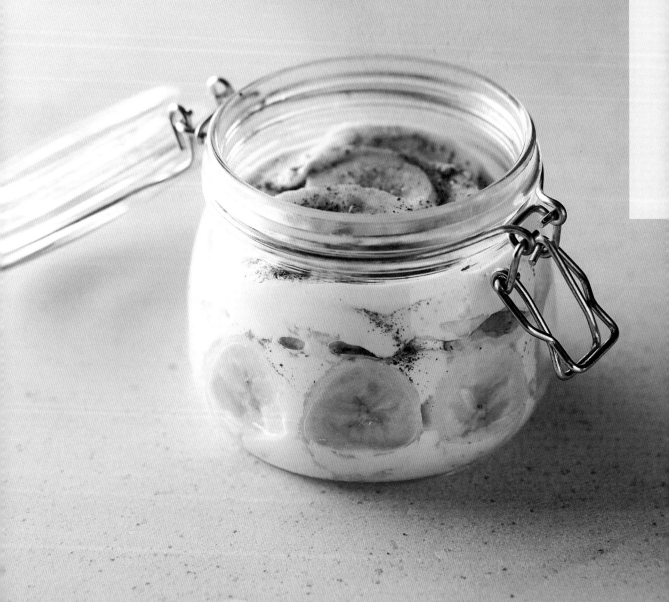

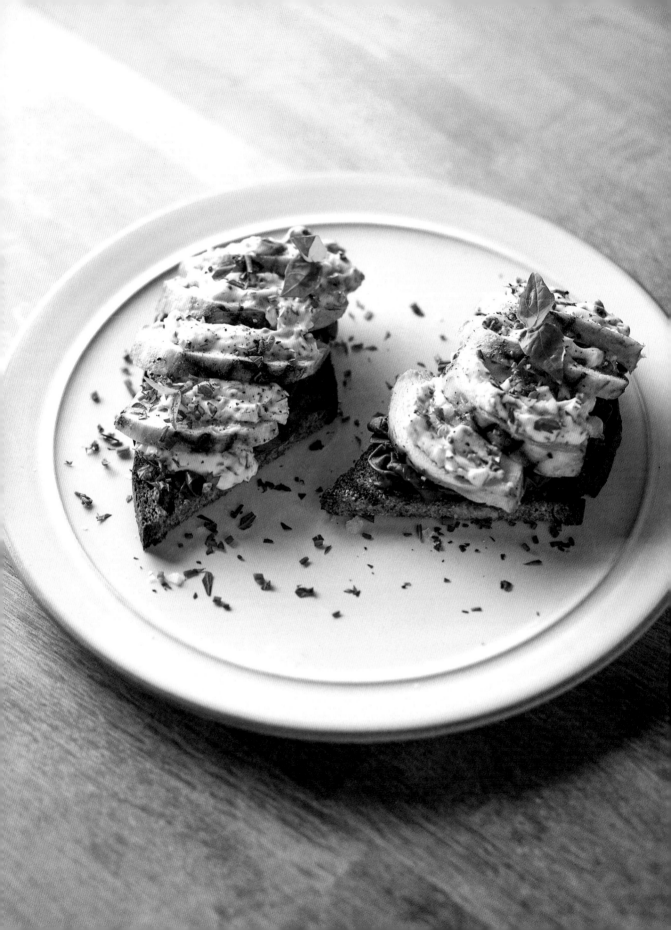

TOAST WITH SPINACH AND CHICKEN IN HERB MAYO

This is a brilliantly simple snack that almost feels like a whole meal in itself. Finish it off with a tasty herby mayo.

1. Heat a skillet and add the sliced chicken. Fry until cooked through, about 10 minutes. Add the spinach leaves for the last 3 minutes to wilt.

2. Meanwhile, mix the mayo with the parsley, basil and chives.

3. Toast the bread, coat the chicken with the herb mayo and serve on toast.

note: slices of bread assume you are using a standard pre-sliced loaf of rye bread. If you are using dense 'pumpernickel' rye bread, use the weights given in brackets rather than slices.

INGREDIENTS	A	B
Chicken breast, sliced	98 g	130 g
Spinach leaves	30 g	40 g
Mayonnaise, reduced fat	1 tbsp	1.5 tbsp
Fresh parsley, finely chopped	2 tsp	3 tsp
Basil leaves, finely chopped	4 leaves	5 leaves
Fresh chives, finely chopped	2 tsp	3 tsp
Rye bread	1.5 slices (68 g)	2.5 slices (90 g)

PROTEIN CARROT CAKE

I've got to say, I do love a carrot cake. To be able to create a great-tasting version which also offers a high protein content makes me very happy!

1. Preheat the oven to 160°C/fan 140°C/gas mark 3. Line and lightly grease a cake tin (any shape, approximately 18cm diameter).

2. In a large bowl, mix together the protein powder, baking powder, carrot and courgette. Add the fresh ginger, stem ginger (this can be substituted for a further 10 g of fresh ginger), raisins, cinnamon, salt and vanilla essence and combine.

3. In a separate bowl, mash the dates with the back of a fork and mix with the milk to make a thin paste. Add to the protein powder mixture.

4. Separate the egg whites into a clean bowl, stirring the yolks into the protein powder mixture. Whisk the egg whites until they form loose peaks then gently fold into the rest of the mixture. Pour the mixture into the prepared cake tin.

5. Bake until a knife comes out clean, about 45 minutes. Remove from the oven and cool for 10 minutes then place on a wire rack to continue to cool. Note: the top will probably collapse a little, but don't worry about this. If you don't like the look of the top of the cake, you can level it with a bread knife.

6. To make the icing: whip the cream cheese with a fork, add the orange zest and slowly add the maple syrup to make a paste. Spread the icing over the cooled cake and decorate with chopped pecan nuts.

7. Cut into 8 slices for A snacks and 6 slices for B snacks and enjoy one piece a day. N. B. you can freeze the sponge before adding the topping to extend the life of the cake.

INGREDIENTS

For the cake

Whey protein	190 g
Baking powder	3 tsp

Carrot, peeled and grated	225 g
Courgette, grated	125 g
Fresh ginger, grated	10 g
Stem ginger (in syrup), finely chopped	25 g
Ground cinnamon	3 tsp
Raisins	55 g
Salt	1 tsp
Vanilla essence	1 tsp
Medjool or other soft dates	170 g
Semi-skimmed milk	140 ml
Eggs	4 small
For the topping	
Fat-free cream cheese	200 g
Orange peel zest	1 orange
Maple syrup	50 g
Pecan nuts	12 g

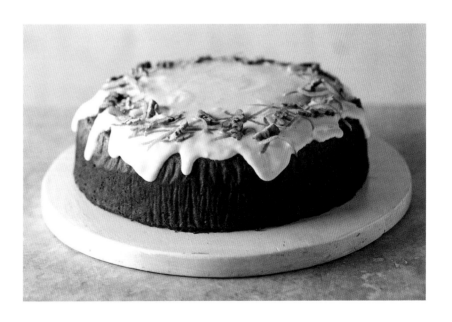

EGG AND POTATO SALAD POT

This simple salad has a lot to offer and always hits the spot, especially with the added mint and lemon juice.

1. Place the new potatoes in a pan of boiling water and simmer for 20–25 minutes, until soft, then drain.

2. Meanwhile, place the eggs in a separate pan of water, bring to the boil and simmer for 7 minutes. Drain, rinse under cold water to cool and peel.

3. Mix together the Skyr yogurt, lemon juice, mint and olive oil, and season with salt and pepper.

4. Toss the potatoes in the dressing and mix in the celery. Ditch all but one egg yolk, chop the remaining egg whites and yolk, and serve on top of the salad.

note: Skyr can be substituted for low-sugar, fat-free Greek yogurt.

INGREDIENTS	A	B
New potatoes, cut into chunks	150 g	200 g
Egg	2 large	3 medium
Skyr natural yogurt	3 tbsp	4 tbsp
Lemon juice	1 tbsp	1 tbsp
Mint, finely chopped	0.5 tbsp	0.5 tbsp
Olive oil	0.5 tsp	1 tsp
Celery, finely chopped	45 g	60 g

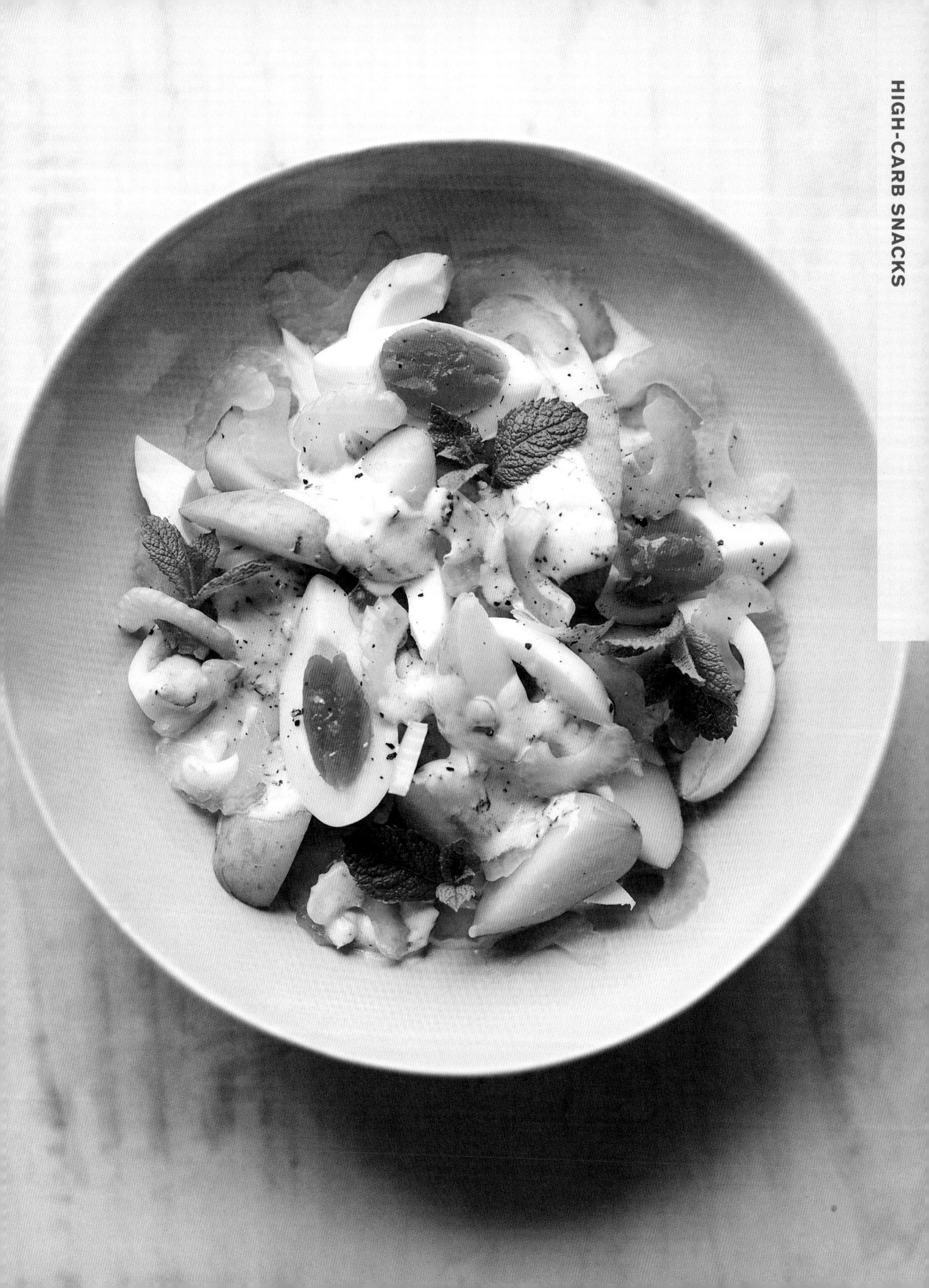

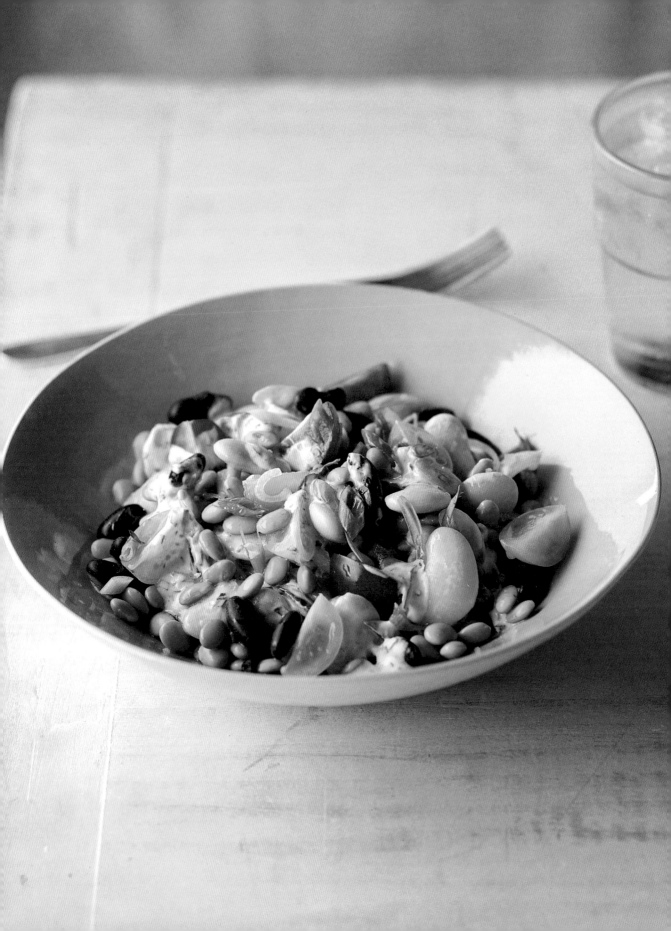

MIXED BEAN SALAD WITH YOGURT

This great little snack is quick and easy to make and could easily be eaten alongside lunch. Maybe even as a starter!

1. In a bowl, stir together the Greek yogurt, Dijon mustard, lemon juice, parsley, tarragon, vinegar and olive oil.

2. Mix with the beans, tomato and spring onions and serve.

note: do not use Greek *style* yogurt instead of Greek yogurt – it often contains much less protein. Make sure the yogurt you use is at least 9g protein per 100g.

INGREDIENTS	A	B
Greek yogurt, 0% fat	75 g	100 g
Dijon mustard	1 tsp	1 tsp
Lemon juice	1 tsp	1 tsp
Parsley, finely chopped	1 tsp	1 tsp
Tarragon, finely chopped	1 tsp	1 tsp
Red wine vinegar	1 tsp	1 tsp
Olive oil	1 tsp	1 tsp
Red kidney beans	68 g	90 g
Butter beans	68 g	90 g
Edamame beans	68 g	90 g
Tomato, chopped	64 g	85 g
Spring onions, finely chopped	15 g	20 g

SWEET POTATO CHIPS WITH TUNA DIP

Sweet potato chips hit the spot for me and using the tuna in the dip is a triumph. Tomato ketchup has nothing on this condiment.

1. Preheat the oven to 200°C/fan 180°C/gas mark 6.

2. Peel and cut the sweet potato into chips and lay on a baking tray. Drizzle over half the olive oil and bake in the oven until the chips are slightly softened but still have a bite, about 30 minutes.

3. Meanwhile, mix the cream cheese, tuna, lemon juice, remaining olive oil and dill in a bowl. Season to taste.

4. Serve the sweet potato chips with the tuna dip.

INGREDIENTS	A	B
Sweet potato	139 g	185 g
Olive oil	1 tsp	1 tsp
Fat-free cream cheese	2.5 tbsp	3 tbsp
Tuna, tinned	94 g	125 g
Lemon juice	1.5 tsp	2 tsp
Dill, finely chopped	1 tsp	1 tsp

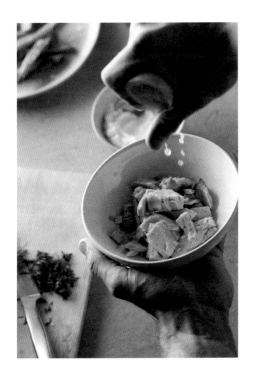
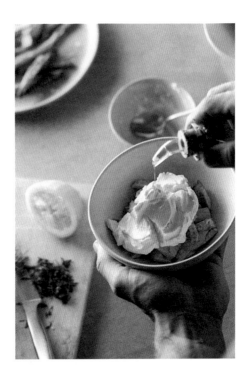
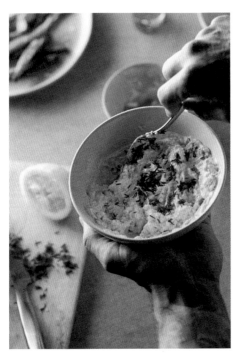
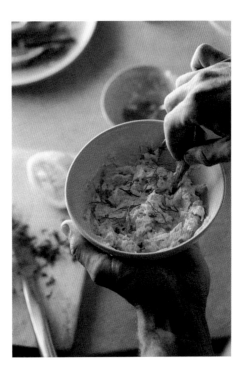

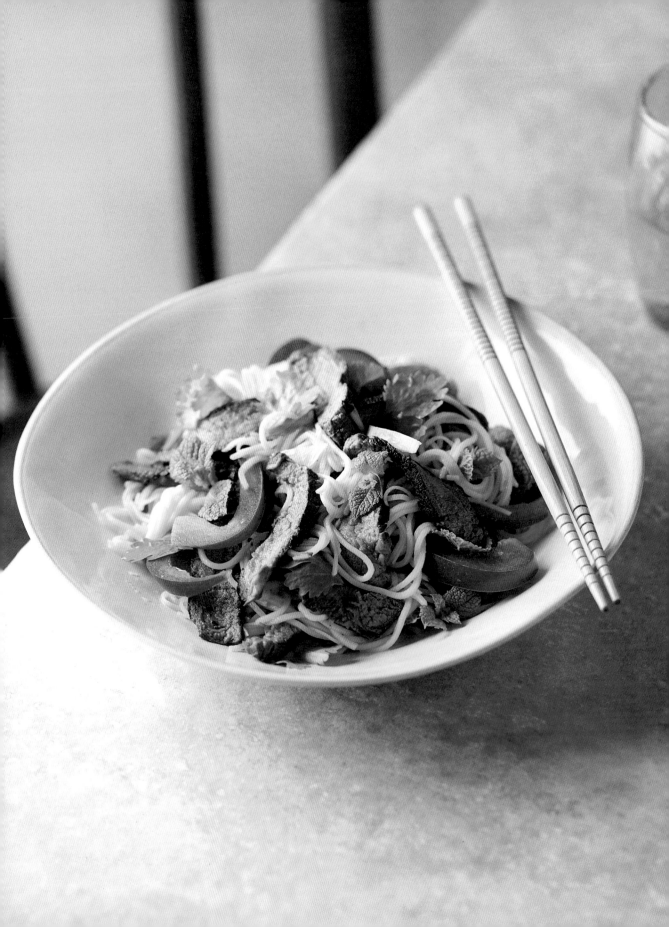

ASIAN NOODLE STEAK SALAD

Of all the snacks, this one is the most satisfying – almost like a mini meal! Big-tasting and quick to make, it can also easily be doubled up for bulk cooking.

1. Heat the sesame oil in a pan, add the sliced beef and fry on high heat until cooked, about 8 minutes.

2. Meanwhile, bring a pan of water to the boil, add the egg noodles and cook until soft, about 5 minutes.

3. Serve the noodles with the beef and sliced red pepper. Dress with the lime juice and sprinkle with chopped mint and coriander.

INGREDIENTS	A	B
Sesame oil	0.5 tsp	0.5 tsp
Beef rump steak, sliced	105 g	140 g
Egg noodles	41 g	55 g
Red pepper, sliced	60 g	80 g
Lime juice	1.5 tsp	2 tsp
Mint, chopped	1 tbsp	1 tbsp
Coriander, chopped	1 tbsp	1 tbsp

SMOKED SALMON, CREAM CHEESE AND CUCUMBER ON RICE CAKES

This snack is so simple to make. I love smoked salmon, and being rich in omega-3, it is also great for your health.

1. Spread the cream cheese on the rice cakes, and top with the cucumber and smoked salmon.

INGREDIENTS	A	B
Fat-free cream cheese	68 g	90 g
Rice cakes	4 cakes	5 cakes
Cucumber, sliced	56 g	75 g
Smoked salmon (hot-smoked)	64 g	85 g

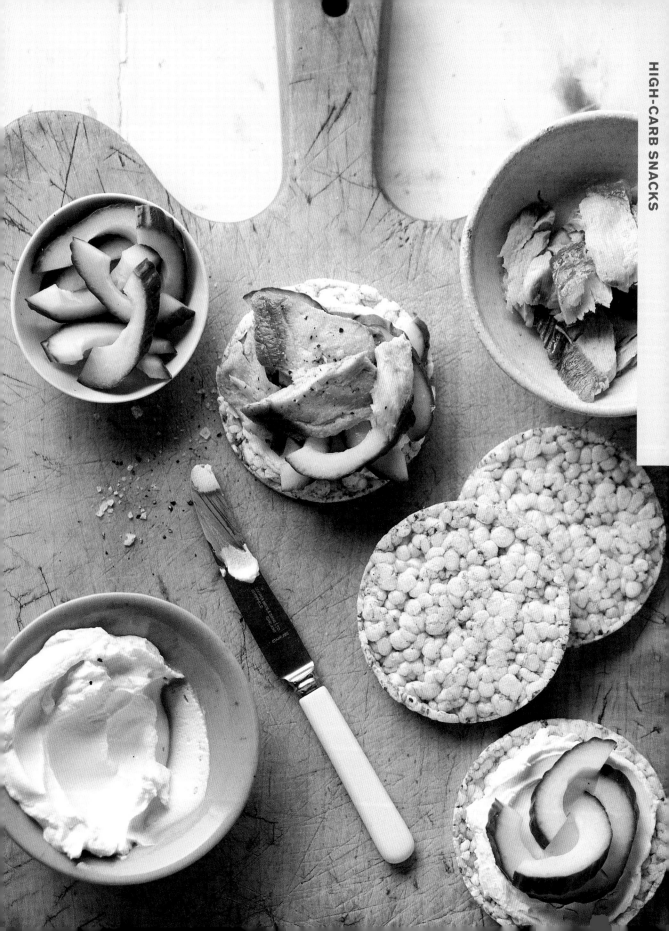

COFFEE AND WALNUT PROTEIN BALLS

This combination of flavours is sensational, making this probably my favourite low-carb snack on the plan. These protein balls are so easy to make and convenient to eat on the move.

1. Mash the dates in a bowl. In a blender, blend the almond flour and walnuts to a powder then mix it together with the whey powder and the dates.

2. Slowly add espresso until the mixture is thick and sticky. Form into balls (see step 3 below) and leave to cool in the fridge before eating.

3. Roll into 4 balls for A snacks and 3 balls for B snacks and enjoy one a day.

INGREDIENTS

Dates, dried	36 g
Almond flour	34 g
Walnuts	70 g
Whey protein	115 g
Shot of brewed espresso	60 ml

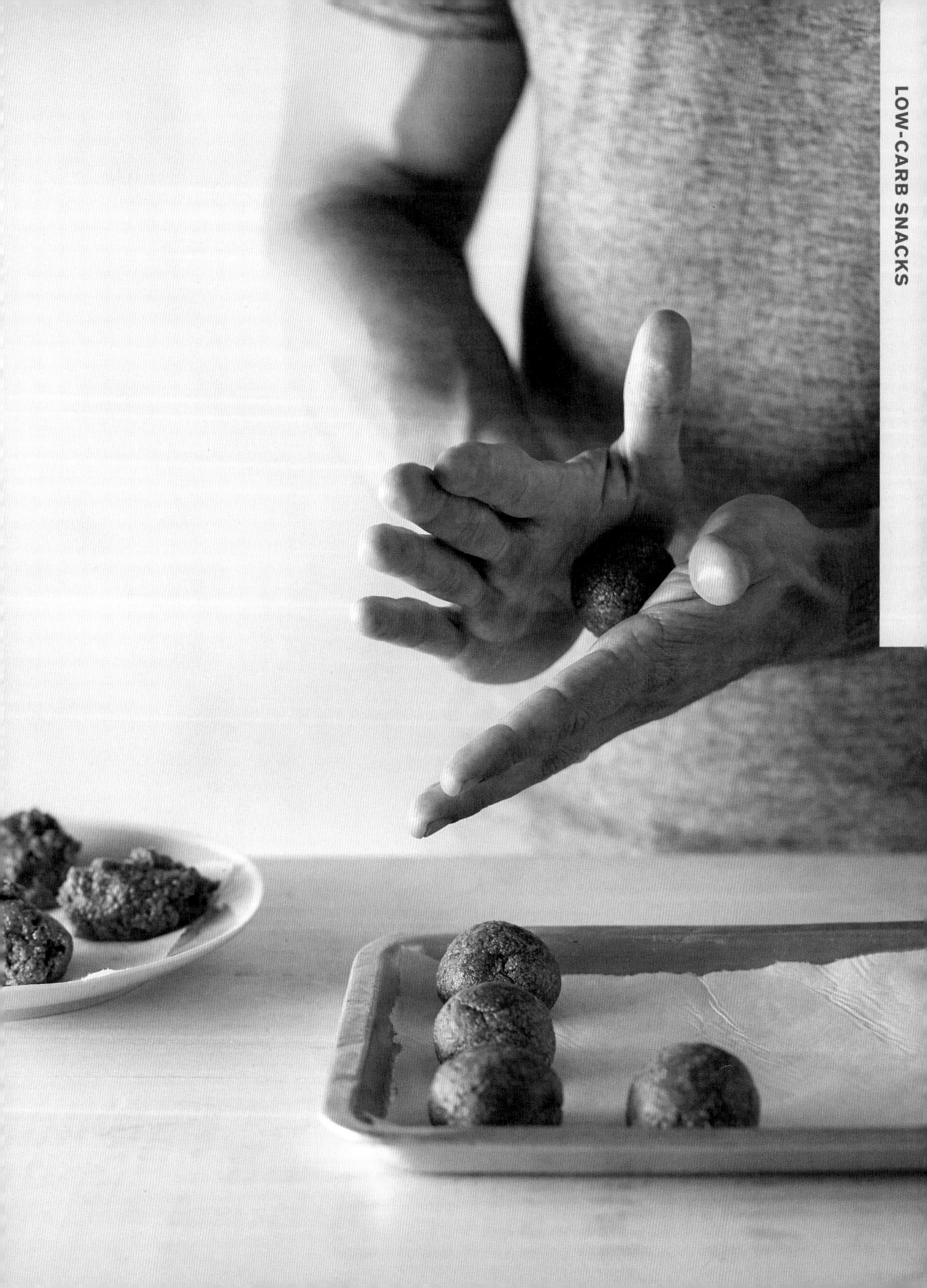

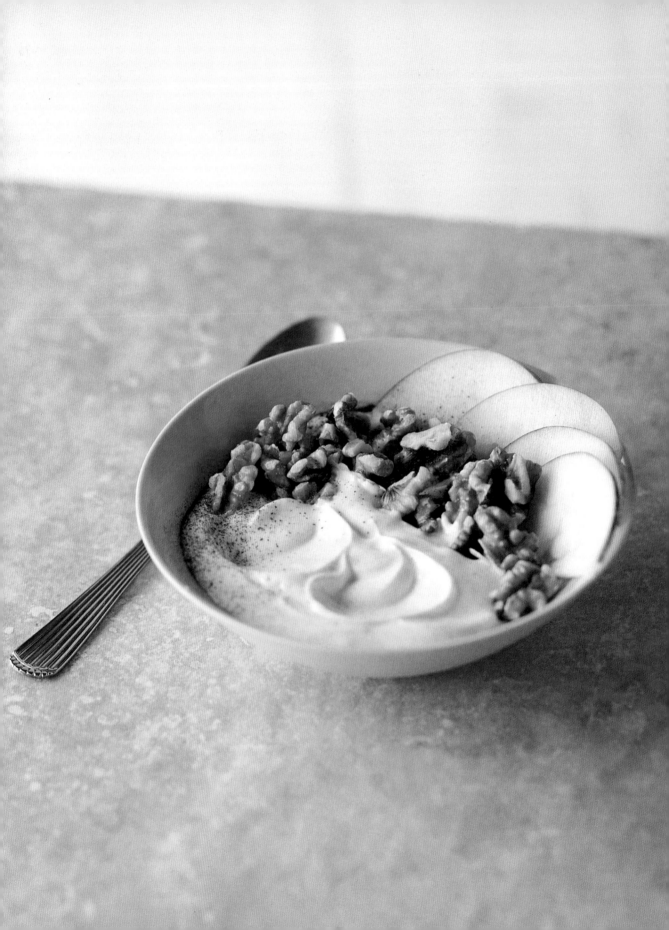

APPLE AND WALNUT WITH VANILLA CINNAMON YOGURT

This snack tastes amazing and keeps those sweet cravings at bay. A perfect pick-me-up at any time of day.

1. Chop the apple and walnuts up finely.

2. Stir into the yogurt, along with the whey powder, cinnamon and vanilla essence. Combine well and serve.

note: Skyr can be substituted for low-sugar, fat-free Greek yogurt.

INGREDIENTS	A	B
Apple	15 g	20 g
Walnuts	23 g	30 g
Skyr natural yogurt	135 g	180 g
Whey protein	12 g	16 g
Ground cinnamon	1 tsp	1 tsp
Vanilla essence	3 drops	4 drops

CINNAMON AND PEANUT BUTTER MUFFINS

More muffins? Yes please! These are deliciously sweet and really fun to bake, making this the perfect afternoon snack.

1. Preheat the oven to 160°C/fan 140°C/gas mark 3. Put the muffin cases in a muffin tray (see step 5 below).

2. Mix the flour, baking powder, bicarbonate of soda, whey powder, cinnamon, peanut butter and a small pinch of salt in a large bowl and mix well.

3. Add the Skyr yogurt, oil and eggs, and stir until well mixed. Leave to stand for a moment, then spoon the mixture into the muffin cases.

4. Bake in the oven for 25 minutes, or until the muffins are well risen and the tops spring back when pressed with a fingertip. Remove from the oven and leave to cool slightly, then transfer to a wire rack.

5. If making A snacks, make eight muffins and eat two muffins per snack; if making B snacks, make nine muffins and eat three muffins per snack.

note: Skyr can be substituted for low-sugar, fat-free Greek yogurt.

INGREDIENTS

Coconut flour	40 g
Baking powder	2 tsp
Bicarbonate of soda	1 tsp
Whey protein	90 g

Ground cinnamon	2 tsp
Peanut butter	35 g
Salt	1 pinch
Skyr natural yogurt	115 g
Vegetable oil	2 tbsp
Eggs	2 medium
Egg white	2 medium

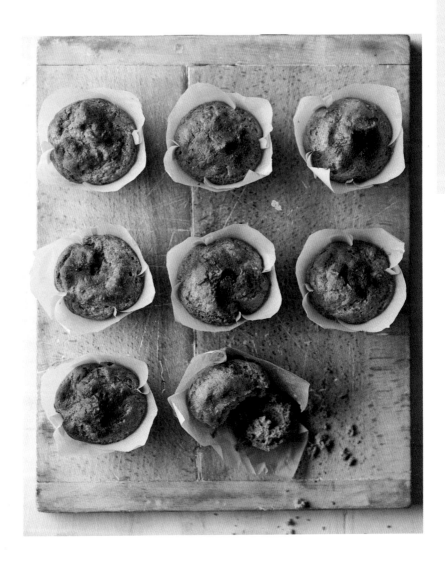

YOGURT AND WHEY

This is a great low-carb option to have alongside lunch as a dessert. And we all know how well pecan and maple syrup go together!

1. Put the pecans in a blender and blend quickly so they are roughly chopped but still retain their texture.

2. In a bowl, stir together the protein powder and the yogurt and add the pecans. Drizzle in the maple syrup and serve.

note: do not use Greek *style* yogurt instead of Greek yogurt – it often contains much less protein. Make sure the yogurt you use is at least 9g protein per 100g.

INGREDIENTS	A	B
Pecan nuts	23 g	30 g
Whey protein	23 g	30 g
Greek yogurt, 0% fat	98 g	130 g
Maple syrup	1 tsp	1 tsp

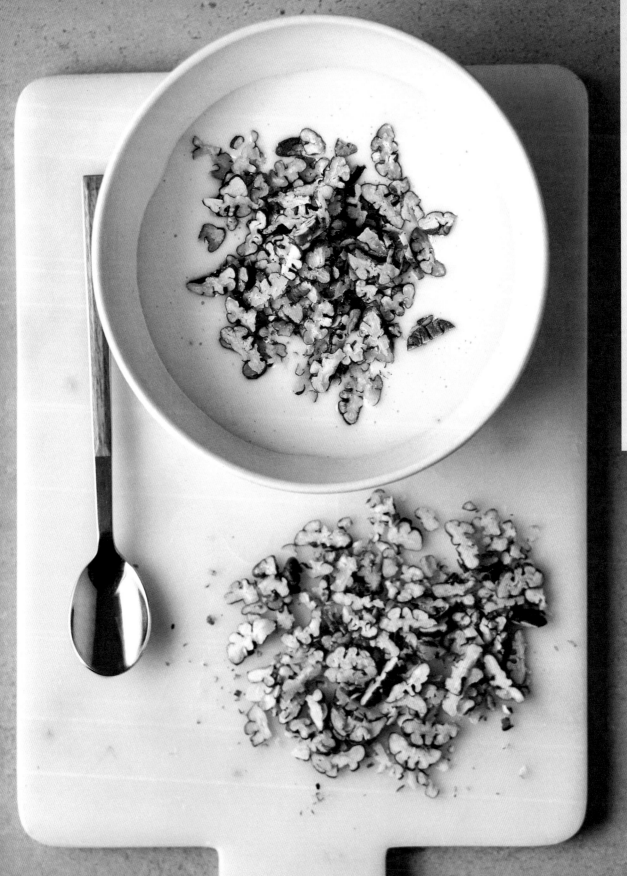

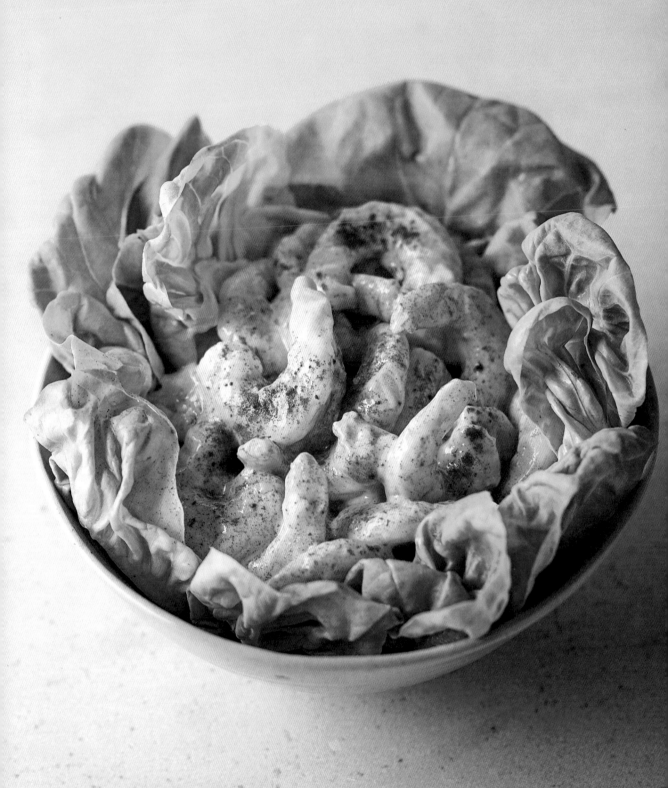

PAPRIKA PRAWN COCKTAIL POT

One of the nation's favourites. The paprika gives a nice little kick as well as being rich in antioxidants: perfect.

1. Mix the ketchup, mayo and paprika together then coat the prawns with the sauce.

2. Serve on a bed of lettuce.

INGREDIENTS	A	B
Tomato ketchup	3.5 tsp	4.5 tsp
Mayonnaise	2.5 tsp	3.5 tsp
Paprika	1 tsp	1 tsp
Cooked prawns	188 g	250 g
Lettuce	60 g	80 g

HONEY YOGURT WITH FLAKED ALMONDS

You can't go far wrong with the delicious mix of honey and nuts. This dish will keep you feeling full and fuelled for the day.

1. Mix the almonds and protein powder into the Skyr yogurt.

2. Serve with a drizzle of honey.

note: Skyr can be substituted for low-sugar, fat-free Greek yogurt.

INGREDIENTS	A	B
Flaked almonds	29 g	38 g
Whey protein	11 g	15 g
Skyr natural yogurt	113 g	150 g
Honey	0.5 tsp	0.5 tsp

AVOCADO AND CHERRY SMOOTHIE

Cherries are known to help with muscle soreness, plus they add a delicious tart flavour that combines well with the avocado. This is a quick and easy smoothie that'll keep you going.

1. Blend all the ingredients together (add extra water if you like your smoothie less thick) and serve.

INGREDIENTS	A	B
Almond milk, unsweetened	113 ml	150 ml
Avocado	71 g	95 g
Skyr natural yogurt	34 g	45 g
Cherries, frozen	7 cherries	9 cherries
Whey protein	26 g	35 g

MATCHA APPLE GREEN SHAKE

This really is a 'super food' shake, which is simple, nutritious and low in carbs. The inclusion of macha green tea powder adds a tiny amount of caffeine, making it the perfect shake to give you a boost. Don't use Greek *style* yogurt instead of Greek yogurt – it often contains less protein. The yogurt needs to have at least 9g protein per 100g.

1. Blend all the ingredients together (add extra water if you like your smoothie less thick) and serve.

INGREDIENTS	A	B
Green apple, grated	23 g	30 g
Almond milk, unsweetened	113 ml	150 ml
Avocado	38 g	51 g
Greek yogurt, 0% fat	34 g	45 g
Whey protein	26 g	34 g
Baby spinach	23 g	30 g
Lime juice	1 tbsp	1 tbsp
Chia seeds	1 tbsp	1 tbsp
Macha green tea powder	1 tsp	1 tsp

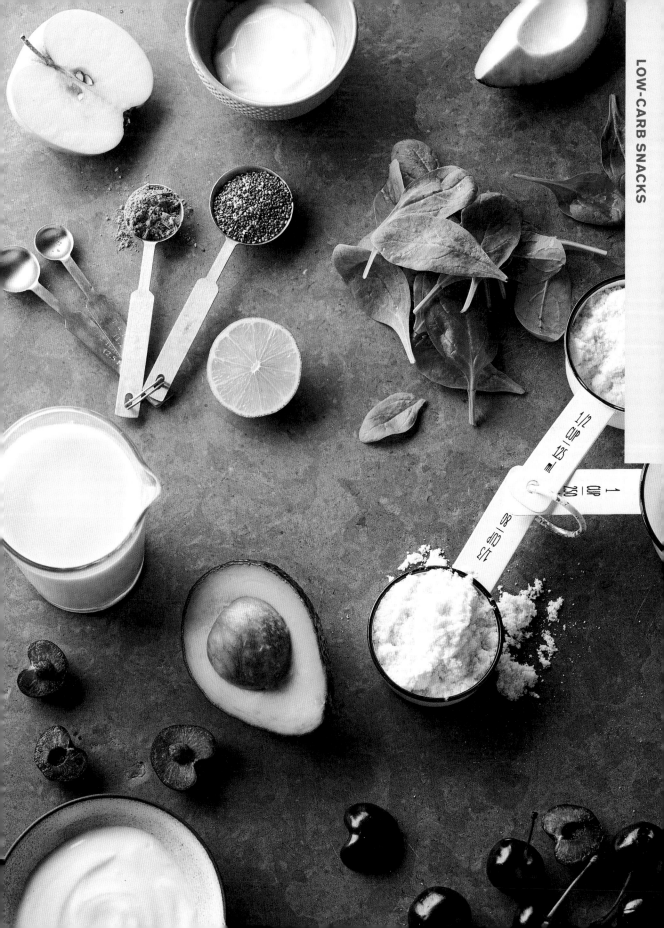

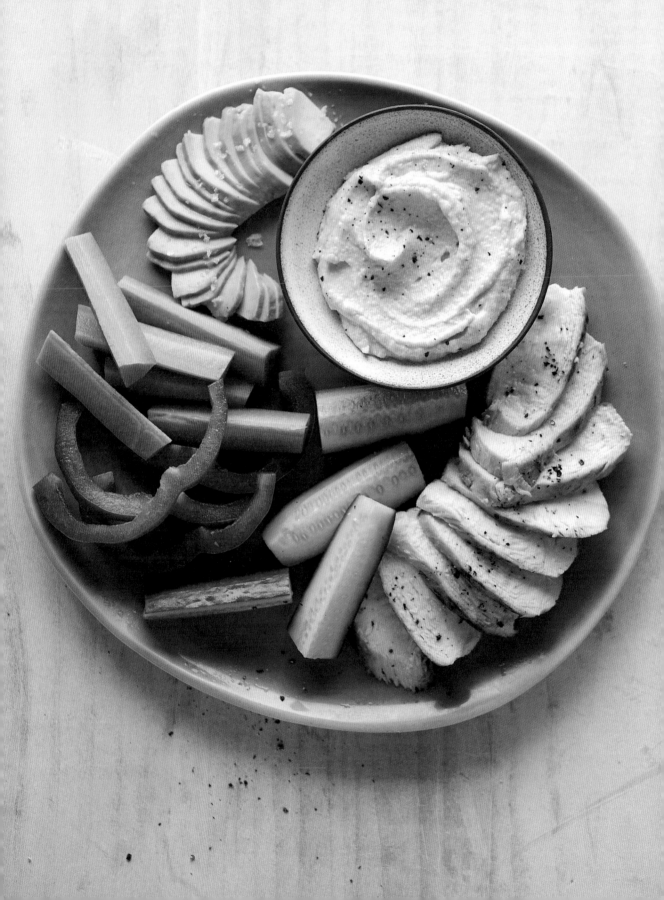

DELI PLATTER WITH HOUMOUS

Chickpeas – the main ingredient in houmous – provide high protein here alongside the chicken. This dish keeps perfectly in the fridge for a few days.

1. Cut the chicken into small chunks, place in a hot non-stick pan and fry for 8–10 minutes until cooked.

2. Meanwhile, cut the red pepper, cucumber and carrot into sticks and slice the avocado.

3. Serve with the chicken and houmous.

INGREDIENTS	A	B
Chicken breast	109 g	145 g
Red pepper	30 g	40 g
Cucumber	56 g	75 g
Carrot, peeled	45 g	60 g
Avocado	26 g	35 g
Houmous	2.5 tbsp	3 tbsp

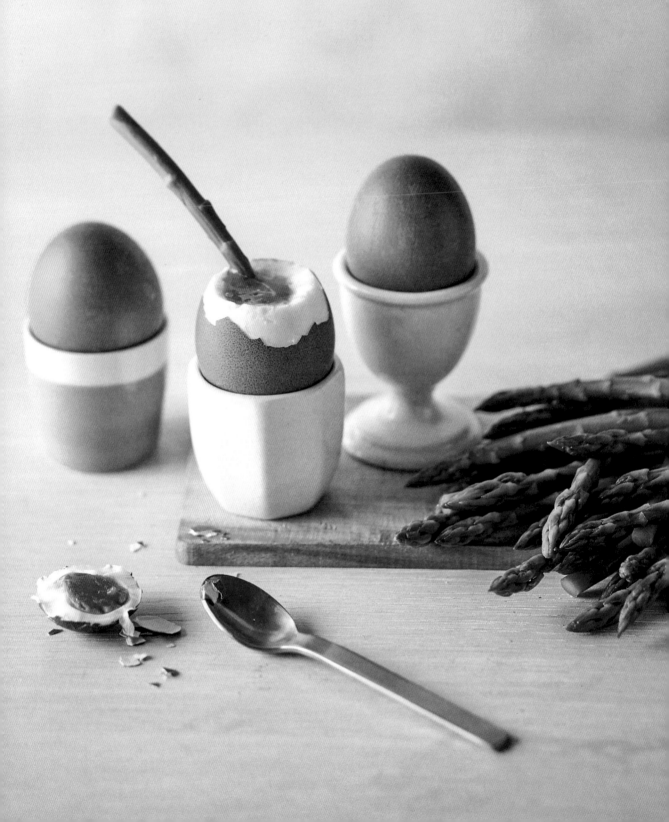

BOILED EGGS AND ASPARAGUS SOLDIERS

Boiled egg with soldiers is an old classic, and replacing bread with asparagus makes for a delicious low-carb twist. The lemony yogurt sauce adds a tasty tang to the flavours.

1. Heat a pan of water. Add the eggs and boil for 5 minutes. Drain and rinse with cold water.

2. Meanwhile, heat a pan, add the oil and fry the asparagus on high for 3 minutes until slightly softened, but still with bite.

3. Mix the yogurt, lemon juice and parsley to make a sauce.

4. Serve the asparagus with your yogurt sauce, and dip in soft-boiled eggs

INGREDIENTS	A	B
Eggs	2 large	3 medium
Asparagus	150 g	200 g
Olive oil	1 tsp	1 tsp
Skyr natural yogurt	2.5 tbsp	3 tbsp
Fresh lemon juice	1 tsp	1 tsp
Fresh parsley	1 tsp	1 tsp

COFFEE AND PROTEIN ICED SHAKE

This is a healthy alternative to the standard coffee-chain drinks. It keeps those wasted calories down by cutting back on the sugar, while still being delicious.

1. In a blender, process the seeds to a fine powder, then add the espresso, whey powder, Greek yogurt and almond milk.

2. Add the ice last and blend to your desired consistency. Add extra water if you like your smoothie less thick.

note: do not use Greek *style* yogurt instead of Greek yogurt - it often contains much less protein. Make sure the yogurt you use is >9g protein per 100g.

INGREDIENTS	A	B
Chia seeds	1 tbsp	1.5 tbsp
Flax seeds	2 tbsp	1 tbsp
Shot of brewed espresso	23 ml	30 ml
Whey protein	24 g	32 g
Greek yogurt, 0% fat	45 g	60 g
Almond milk, unsweetened	98 ml	130 ml
Ice	38 g	50 g

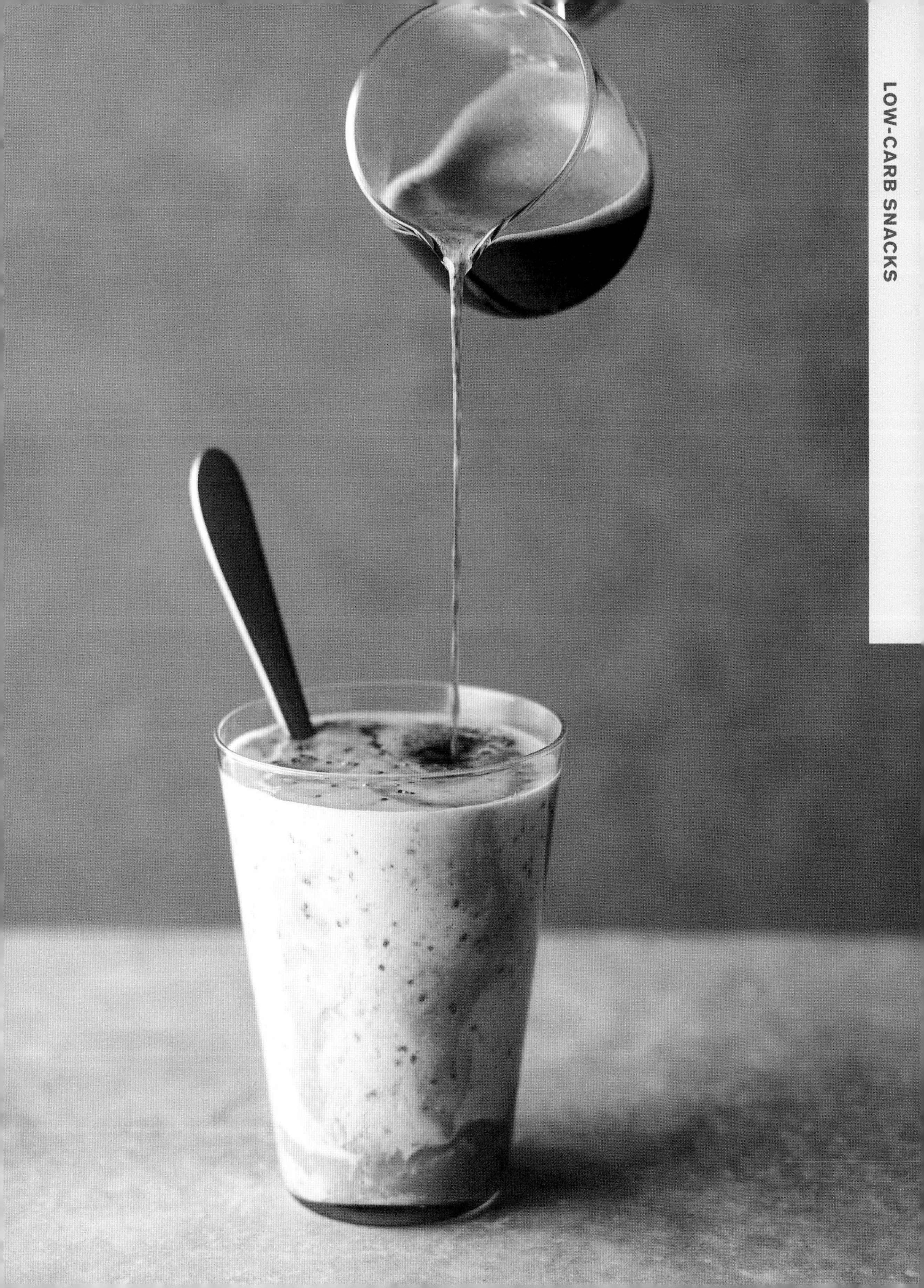

SIMPLE CINNAMON PEANUT PROTEIN SHAKE

This protein shake is always a go-to after a tiring session at the gym or a busy day filled with meetings. It makes sure you get what you need on the go. The peanut butter and cinnamon adds something a little different and tastes great.

1. Blend all the ingredients together (add extra water if you like your smoothie less thick) and serve.

INGREDIENTS	A	B
Almond milk, unsweetened	113 ml	150 ml
Whey protein	26 g	35 g
Peanut butter	1.5 tbsp	2 tbsp
Cinnamon	1 tsp	1 tsp

HAM, EGG AND AVOCADO WITH HONEY MUSTARD

This is a low-carb approach to eating, combining protein from the eggs and the fats from the avocado – all enhanced with a subtle kick of mustard.

1. Bring a pan of water to the boil, add the eggs and boil for 7 minutes. Drain and rinse with cold water to cool.

2. In a small bowl, mix the mustard and honey well. Dice the ham and the egg and serve with the sliced avocado and the mustard dressing.

INGREDIENTS	A	B
Eggs	2 small	2 medium
English mustard	1.5 tsp	2 tsp
Honey	1 tsp	1 tsp
Ham	98 g	130 g
Avocado, sliced	26 g	35 g

MOZZARELLA, HAM AND TOMATOES WITH MEDITERRANEAN DRIZZLE

Having spent many years visiting Italy I had to incorporate this classic combo in the book. It will bring the taste of Italy to your kitchen.

1. In a small bowl, mix together the olive oil, vinegar, honey, Dijon mustard, basil and garlic powder.

2. Arrange the slices of mozzarella, tomato and ham on a plate and drizzle with the dressing.

INGREDIENTS	A	B
Extra virgin olive oil	1 tsp	1 tsp
Red wine vinegar	1 tsp	1 tsp
Honey	0.5 tsp	0.5 tsp
Dijon mustard	0.5 tsp	0.5 tsp
Basil, finely chopped	4 leaves	5 leaves
Garlic powder	1 pinch	1 pinch
Low-fat mozzarella, sliced	30 g	40 g
Tomatoes, sliced	98 g	130 g
Parma ham, sliced	90 g	120 g

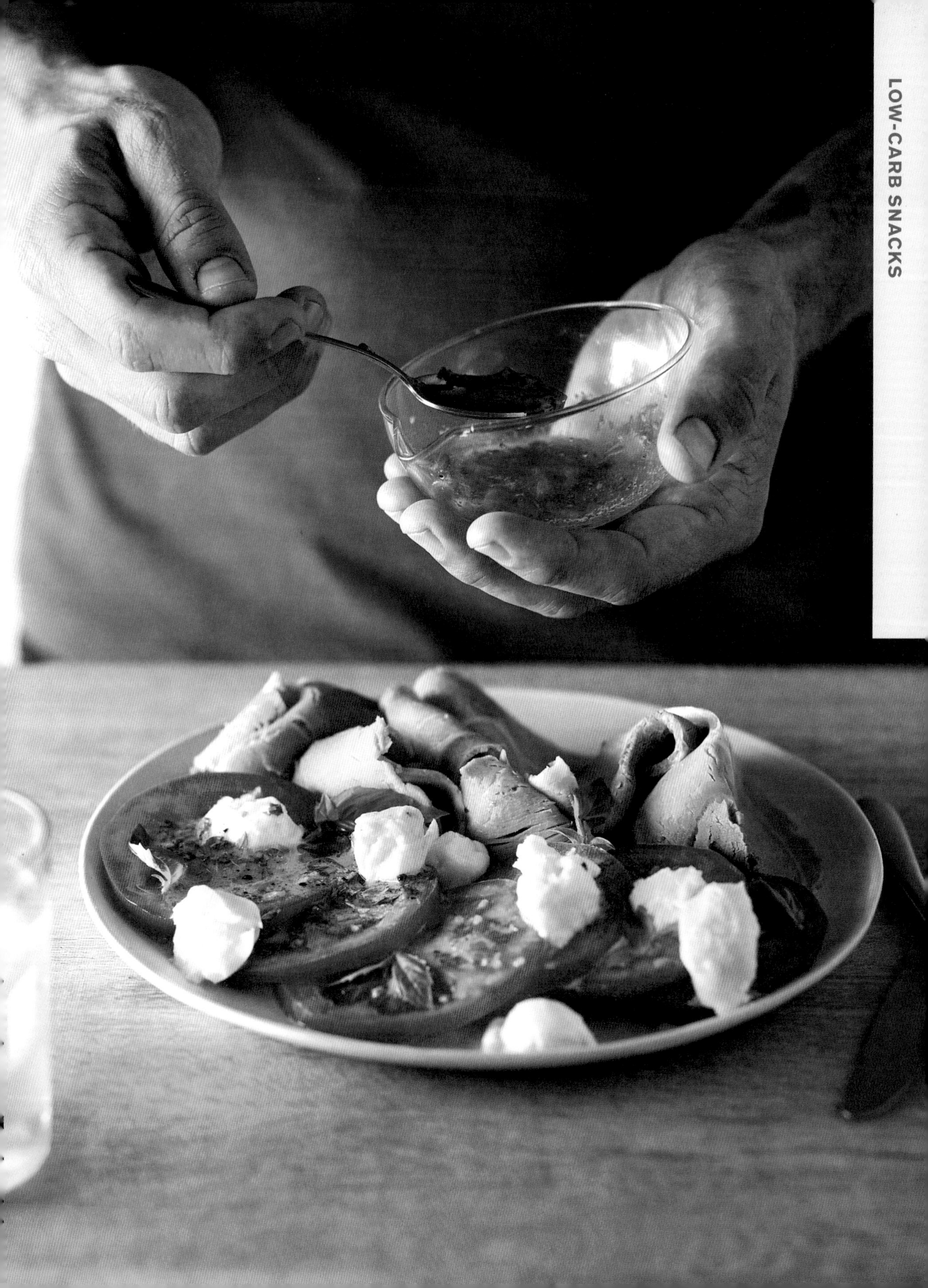

CASE STUDY: **JOSH**

Now I'm going to hand over to Josh, 34, who, like so many people, has tried a number of exercise regimes but struggled to find a long-term solution. What makes me very happy is how easy he found the plan to incorporate into his busy life, meaning he can continue to follow it for a long time to come.

Weight lost: 29lbs / 13kg
Exercise per week: 5+ hours
Calories per day: 2,000–2,200 calories
Reason for starting: To see abs, to feel confident enough to take off my shirt – and to look the way I feel on the inside on the outside.

Have you tried losing weight before?
Yes, I've tried many different exercise plans, but found that some weren't sustainable. With some I lacked energy because of low-carb meal plans, or, on the flip side, the calories were too high so I never saw the results I desired. None of them were personalised to my needs.

How did you feel when you started the plan?
I was unhappy about my appearance and the example I was providing to my kids. I had fallen into bad habits – I had newborns so I was putting them before myself without knowing how simple it could be if someone did the planning for me.

How do you feel now?
I feel confident! I have proven to myself that dedication and consistency is key to achieving the results you are looking for.

What did you like the most in terms of following the plan?
Tracking macros and weight on your own isn't practical when all of life's stresses are in front of you. David's plans calculated that all for me and being able to pick recipes

and prepare them in advance saved a lot of time and actually gave me more time to focus on the more important things without having the added stress.

What exercises did you like the most or find gave you the most results?
I enjoyed seeing my weights numbers go up, but I wouldn't say there was a particular exercise that gave the most results. The whole programme pieced together the look I wanted and is something I could keep following for a healthy lifestyle for a long time to come.

Was there anything you found tricky?
I can't say I disliked anything. I will say coming from consuming around 3000-3500 calories to 2000 was difficult for the first 10 days. I found drinking extra liquids, trying to push breakfast later into the day and maintaining a shorter eating window was helpful if I wasn't training first thing in the morning.

Will you keep going with the plan now?
Yes of course. I want to be more muscular and be even leaner for next summer!

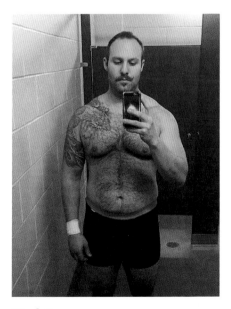

Week 1

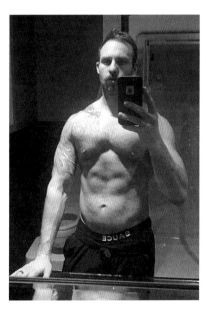

Week 8

PART 3:
MOVEMENT

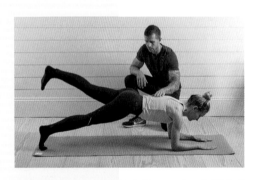

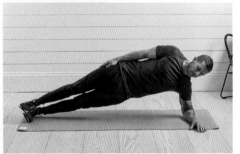

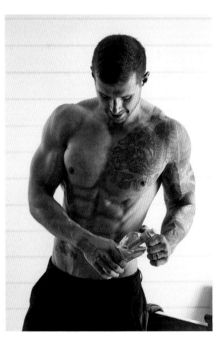

CHOOSING YOUR TRAINING PLANS

We've finally reached that point. That life-changing moment where your health and fitness is going to improve forever.

To lose body fat and become fitter and healthier, movement is essential. You can achieve results without it, but the more you move, the more results you're likely to see – including changes in your body composition and improved health. Adding movement also allows you to eat more food – great news! – and still make progress. I would always encourage more than three hours of movement each week for health reasons, but results are possible no matter how much time you have – the key is eating the right number of calories for your level of activity.

TYPES OF TRAINING

There are two main types of movement: resistance training and cardio – I don't believe you should put all your eggs in one basket when it comes to the type of exercise you do. They both serve a purpose and help to provide variety. In addition, there is circuit training, which is a combination of resistance and cardio.

#1: RESISTANCE (OR WEIGHT) TRAINING (PAGES 198–249) Arguably the most important exercise you can do, resistance training is a bit like running in a swimming pool. You can't run as fast as you can on land, because you're working against the water. This resistance means your muscles have to work that much harder to move you along. But you don't need to be in a pool to make it work for you! Resistance training only needs a force to resist your movements. In a gym environment, this is usually done by weights, but you can also do it at home using hand weights (you can buy these for under £10) or just focus on exercises that

use your own bodyweight instead (e.g. push-ups). In this plan I have included both options – a gym-based plan that uses weights, and a home-based plan that uses bodyweight, but I would recommend investing in weights even if you do the latter: they will allow you to adjust the level of resistance with ease so you can progress when you need to, and also step back and reduce the resistance when you need to.

The use of resistance training is crucial to a healthy lifestyle and will make your fat-loss journey much easier and more sustainable than if you choose to take this journey without it. Second to getting your calories under control, adding weights to your plan is just about the smartest thing you can do.

THE MANY BENEFITS OF RESISTANCE TRAINING

- **It improves insulin sensitivity:** The high demands of resistance training will encourage blood sugar to your muscles rather than fat cells. This process of high demand will remain even after your workout has finished. Having more lean muscle will encourage your body to be more sensitive to insulin and utilise carbohydrates more effectively.

- **It reduces the risk of injury:** Strength training can increase bone density, improve your balance and helps with your physical stability. Providing your form is right when exercising, you can limit the risk of injuries that might derail your efforts. As we age, we all begin to lose muscle and bone mass. By regularly undertaking resistance training, your muscles will begin to adapt to the stresses the weights place upon your body by becoming bigger and stronger, protecting you from the onset of osteoporosis.

- **It enhances your mood:** Anaerobic exercises, like weight lifting, have a positive effect on mood.

- **It gives you the EPOC effect:** EPOC – Excess Post-exercise Oxygen Consumption – basically means an increased rate of oxygen intake following strenuous activity. During recovery from exercise, we need extra oxygen to restore the body to a resting state and adapt it to the exercise just performed.

#2: CARDIO (PAGES 250–253)

Cardio: some people love it; other people hate it. Cardio is classed as any movement that gets your heart rate up and increases your blood circulation, like running, power walking, cycling and swimming. For most people, cardio is a way to burn those excess calories.

One type of cardio we'll be using is **LISS or Low-Intensity Steady State** cardio, which involves cardio exercises that are performed over relatively prolonged periods, generally up to one hour, at a low intensity. This could be a brisk walk on the treadmill, or a slow pedal on the spin bike. Don't think because it's low intensity it isn't effective: **LISS** works by increasing your heart rate into a targeted 'fat-loss' zone and keeping it there.

Another type of cardio I use is **interval training**, which essentially means bursts of intense work followed by rest periods. I say 'rest', but don't think you'll be sitting around doing nothing! Some interval training routines will recommend a complete rest period, but in general the training will be more effective if you keep moving, just at a slower pace.

EXTRA: CIRCUIT TRAINING (PAGE 254)

This is a one-stop training session, combining both resistance and cardiovascular exercises, moving quickly between several different exercises. Circuit training is designed to keep your heart rate and pulse high, while working all muscle groups. Because the rest periods are kept very short in circuit training, these exercises put a high demand on your body, depleting your energy stores and boosting fat burning after the session.

HOW TO STRETCH

Keeping flexible will help keep you moving and limit the risk of injuries, aches and pains associated with tight muscle. This section will provide you with a stretching routine that will work through all the major muscle groups.

STRETCHES

It is important to reiterate that static stretching before training or athletic performance may not be beneficial, and may cause injury. Make sure you perform static stretching **after** your workout when you are warmed up. Here are some other stretching tips:

- ☐ Stretch to just before the point of discomfort
- ☐ Keep breathing during the stretch. Avoid breath holding
- ☐ Aim to hold each stretch for 10–20 seconds
- ☐ If you feel pain, stop the stretch
- ☐ Complete 2–3 repeats of each stretch before starting the next stretch

UPPER BODY STRETCHES

STANDING PEC STRETCH

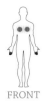

FRONT

Begin standing upright with your forearm against a wall or door frame. Keep your elbow bent to 90 degrees. Turn your body away from the wall until you feel a stretch across your chest. Repeat for the other side.

KNEELING LAT STRETCH

BACK

Start in a kneeling position with a bench in front of you with your knees and feet hip-width apart. Lean forwards and place your hand on the bench. Keep your arm straight. There should be a straight line from the shoulders, through the elbows to the wrists. The other hand remains on the floor directly below the shoulder. Lean into the side with the arm extended on the bench to get the stretch. Repeat for the other side.

TRICEPS STRETCH

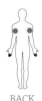

BACK

Place one hand behind your neck with your elbow in the air. Place your other hand on your elbow and gently pull towards your head. Hold and repeat with your other arm. Repeat for the other side.

LOWER BODY STRETCHES

GLUTE STRETCH

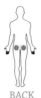

BACK

Start in a seated position with your right leg on the floor. Bend your left leg and place your left foot over your right leg. Place your right arm over your left leg so your elbow can be used to push the left knee and stretch. Hold and repeat for the other side.

STANDING QUADRICEPS STRETCH

FRONT

Standing on one foot, lift the bottom of the raised leg (just above the ankle). Pull your heel into your bum and push the hips forwards with your body in an upright position. Hold and repeat on the other side. Lean your other arm on a wall or table if you feel unbalanced.

SINGLE LEG HAMSTRING STRETCH

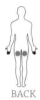

BACK

Start in a seated position on the floor. Place one leg out straight in front and bend the other leg so it is flat to the floor with your foot up against the inside of your thigh. Bend forward from the waist. Aim to keep your back flat. Hold and repeat with the other leg.

STANDING CALF STRETCH

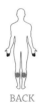

BACK

Place one foot in front of the other about 18 inches apart. Keep your back leg straight and heel on the floor and lean forwards to feel the calf stretch, bending the front leg as needed. You can also push against a wall to increase the intensity of the stretch. Hold and repeat with the other leg.

KNEELING HIP FLEXOR STRETCH

FRONT

Start in a kneeling position then lunge forward with one leg. Place hands on front knee and keep your body upright and lean forward to get a stretch in the hip. Hold the stretch. Repeat with other side.

STAY SAFE

If you are suffering from any pre-existing injuries or conditions prior to starting your plan, it is important to get clearance from your doctor to allow you to begin. There may be certain exercises that you cannot do based on those existing injuries. If that's the case, then please ensure you adapt your plan accordingly. If you are unsure of what movements you can or can't do, then I suggest working through the movements with an exercise professional (e.g. an instructor at your gym) prior to starting your plan. This will ensure you do the movements safely and effectively. The last thing either of us wants is for you to get injured, so let's try and mitigate that risk as much as we can. Here are my top tips for exercising safely:

#1 MAKE SURE YOU WARM UP THOROUGHLY The reason we warm up is to bring blood to the muscle you're about to train, so that your body temperature gets warmer, making your muscles more supple and supporting free and coordinated movement. I've seen far too many people statically stretch their calves once for about 5 seconds before starting a run. This kind of warm-up can actually cause injury: stretching has an analgesic or painkilling effect, which makes you less sensitive to warning signs from your body that you may be risking injury. It can also impede speed and strength and increase risk because of the cellular damage it can cause to the muscle.

Start with a general warm-up of 5 minutes of cardio exercise to bring up blood flow and body temperature. When doing the resistance plans, you need to warm the specific muscle (or muscle group). I suggest 3–4 sets of 8–12 reps of the movements you're going to be doing (if you're not sure what sets and reps are, flick to page 198), starting without any weight at all then progressively increasing the resistance until you reach your desired set weight. When moving into the next exercise, your body may be warm, but I suggest performing another warm-up set prior to the next full-effort set. This will reduce the risk of injury.

#2 PRACTICE GOOD FORM
The way you move weights, the way you position yourself while doing so and the movements you undertake in resistance training or cardio all make up your form. Bad form can result in injury. Make sure you read through all my guidance on how to perform each exercise thoroughly before you begin. If there is anything you're unsure about, please look at my website or speak to a fitness professional about it. Just like with driving, it's natural that bad habits may creep in over time, so be mindful of what you're doing, and how you're doing it, over time.

#3 WORK TO YOUR ABILITY
We all have limits. As much as you'd like to lift the heaviest weights, run the furthest or burpee with the best of them, your current fitness levels might mean that's not possible. You'll get there, but I want you to get there without hurting yourself. If you're trying to lift more weight than you can handle, then injury is going to occur. Use weights you can manage, build up distance and speed in cardio gradually and increase the resistance or intensity when you feel able to.

If you set the bar or dumbbell with more weight than you can safely lift, then the danger of literally dropping the weight on yourself is very real. It could also cause problems for your muscles and joints, tendons and ligaments as they struggle to stabilise your limbs as you lift without control and with poor form. As a rule of thumb, if you can't lift the full number of reps specified, then you're using too much weight. There's no problem in reducing the weight to reduce the risk of injury. It is important to have full control of your movements as you exercise.

#4 PUSH YOURSELF – BUT NOT THROUGH PAIN
If you're exercising and start to feel pain, then stop doing it. Don't just 'push through it'. The pain you're feeling is a warning sign from your body that something is wrong. If you ignore it, then it will soon become more serious, potentially scuppering your entire plan. It is quite common to feel a little stiff before you exercise, a feeling that can be relieved by warming up properly. But if the pain doesn't go, or gets worse, then seek medical attention. If you suffer from a prior injury, or pick up an injury then it's not the end of the world, or even the plan necessarily. Make an appointment to see a doctor or exercise professional to determine what you can and cannot do.

YOUR WEEKLY MOVEMENT

Your training plan will depend on the amount of exercise you're able to do per week. You'll see that the resistance plans are the foundation for each level – how much interval, circuit and L.I.S.S training you want to add on top of that is up to you.

LEVEL 1: 1–3 HOURS PER WEEK

☐ At least one session from the Resistance Training: Home-based Plan (page 198) or at least one Level 1 session from the Gym-based Plan (page 227)

☐ Optional interval session (page 252) or 30–40 mins of LISS (page 250).

LEVEL 2: 3–5 HOURS PER WEEK

☐ At least two sessions from the Resistance Training: Home-based Plan (page 198) or at least two Level 2 sessions from the Gym-based Plan (page 227)

☐ One interval session (page 252) and 30-40 mins of LISS (page 250).

LEVEL 3: 5+ HOURS PER WEEK

☐ All three sessions from the Resistance Training: Home-based Plan (page 198) or all three Level 3 sessions from the Gym-based Plan (page 227)

☐ Two interval sessions (page 252) that include 40–60 mins LISS (page 250).

☐ One circuit training (page 254).

N.B. 5–7 hours of activity is the optimal amount at Level 3. I wouldn't suggest much more unless you are training for a specific sport or event (e.g. like an iron man).

PROGRESSION: HOW YOU'LL GET STRONGER AND FITTER

Let me introduce you to someone: meet Milo of Croton. Milo wanted to become the greatest wrestler in Ancient Greece and win six Olympic laurels. To do that, Milo had to train like the rest of us, but his method was a little unorthodox: he borrowed a newborn calf and he carried it, every day. As the calf grew, so did Milo's strength – until he he could carry the now fully grown bull upon his back.

This isn't a history lesson, I promise! The lesson is, to get stronger, you must continually make your muscles work harder than they're used to. As a rule of thumb, 'If it's easy, make it harder.' (That's 'harder', not impossible! Pushing yourself to extremes is never going to work.) With weight or resistance training you can do this by increasing the weight you're lifting, then the number of sets you're doing. With cardio training, you can increase the length of time you spend doing it, or up the intensity. And for circuit training you can increase the weights or intensity, lengthen the session, or gradually decrease the rest periods between each exercise.

Improvements in strength and fitness are not linear however, eventually your gains in strength will plateau. To overcome this plateau, you'll find my resistance training plans provide variations in movements to provide a new stimulus.

FAQS

Q: HOW MUCH TIME SHOULD I SPEND EXERCISING IN EACH SESSION?

A: It depends on which sessions you are doing, but they could be anything from 20 through to 75 minutes; it's up to you and dependent on how much time you have to give.

Q: IS THERE AN OPTIMUM TIME TO TRAIN? DO YOU LOSE MORE FAT IF YOU TRAIN AFTER FASTING?

A: Don't worry about any of this! Focus on simply getting your activity in at the most convenient time for you. The pros and cons on training time are exaggerated; the most important thing is simply getting it done consistently. By working it into your day and not working your day around it, your exercise routine will become much more sustainable.

Q: ARE REST DAYS CHEATING?

A: No. Resting, or having a rest day, is far too often overlooked – it plays a crucial part in any credible fitness plan. In the decade and more that I've been a personal trainer, I've rarely seen a schedule or plan that would be made worse by including a rest within it. If anything, regular rest periods will help you succeed, as including rest days helps prevent overuse of your joints and muscles that can occur when pushing too hard without having a break. When it comes to recovery, resting also gives your muscles the time they need to grow. Let's not forget that when you're exercising, you're effectively tearing the fibre of the muscle so that it can repair itself and come back bigger and stronger. That only happens with rest. Continuing to work on it in the gym isn't going to make that happen.

When most people hear 'rest' they think immediately of 'sleep', which is fine because sleep is another part of your plan that needs to work well to achieve your results. One of the problems with overtraining is that training too hard can put your body in a state of restlessness, making getting a good night's sleep difficult. By including a rest day (or days), your body will withdraw from a state of readiness and your heart rate will reduce, allowing a good night's sleep.

Regardless of your experience, I recommend including a bare minimum of 2 rest days per week from resistance work or high intensity exercise, to allow your body to recover (more if you are new to exercising regularly). On these days, you can do low intensity exercise if you want.

Q: DO I NEED TO BE IN A GYM TO DO THESE EXERCISES?

A: Not everyone is able – or wants – to use a gym, and that's fine. Instead you can focus on your bodyweight resistance sessions as a priority, or invest in your own set of weights. You can buy them cheaply online, especially if they're second-hand.

Q: WILL WEIGHT LIFTING MAKE ME BULKY?

A: This is a misconception. I often hear 'I don't want to look like a bodybuilder', to which I reply, 'Thank goodness for that!' Looking like a bodybuilder doesn't happen by accident. These men and women didn't just do some weights one day and wake up the next looking like that. It takes years of effort specifically focused on achieving this task. Your plan is not focused on this: it's focused on fat-loss and toning.

Q: WHAT WEIGHTS SHOULD I BE USING?

A: The heaviest weight you can lift safely, with full control, for the designated number of reps. If you are able to lift more reps than prescribed then you should increase the weight.

Q: WHAT TYPE OF CARDIO IS BEST?

A: I don't believe in comparing exercises as they all have certain benefits for certain goals. Interval training is high intensity and will burn a lot of calories in a short time. L.I.S.S. is low impact and optimised to burn fat for fuel, so it is less effort but you will burn fewer calories in the same time period. Ultimately the purpose of cardio, in addition to improving health and fitness, is to burn calories, so provided your calorie intake is correct, they will both be effective for fat loss.

Q: WILL I GET INJURED DOING ANY OF THIS TRAINING?

A: All exercise and movement comes with some risk. You can reduce these risks with thorough warm-ups and using good form on your movements. See pages 185–189 for more information.

Q: I HAVE A PRE-EXISTING INJURY – CAN I STILL DO THE PLAN?

A: You will need to check with your doctor or an exercise professional to determine whether you can follow the plan safely.

Q: WHAT WILL HAPPEN TO MY MUSCLES IF I STOP TRAINING? WILL THEY BECOME FLABBY?

A: If you stop using your muscles, of course they'll eventually decrease in strength and size. I often get asked if your muscle will turn to fat. Don't worry, this isn't possible, muscle will not turn to fat if you stop using it. However, I would encourage you to continue to use your muscle for the rest of your life. Losing muscle will have a long-term negative effect on your body composition, health and fat loss.

FINAL TOP TIPS

- Focus on resistance first.

- Try to space your resistance sessions out throughout the week rather than doing them over consecutive days.

- Add LISS., circuits and intervals to bring your hours up.

- If you suffer from muscle soreness and fatigue then LISS is a good low-impact option.

- If your time is restricted then adding some intervals will be beneficial.

- If you are unable to perform movements then get advice on alternatives.

- If you are very overweight, then using just LISS for the first few weeks may be beneficial to drop some weight before starting resistance movements if these are too challenging at your current weight.

- Feel free to include classes and activities you enjoy on top of your resistance sessions if you have the time within your level.

- Enjoy it. Rope in a friend or find someone you can work out with. Exercising with friends is more enjoyable and will increase accountability!

- Get support. The online #TeamKingsbury community is here for you. If you need advice, support or encouragement, we've got you.

CASE STUDY: **MATT**

Next up is Matt. Matt struggled to find an exercise regime that he could fit into his busy life. Using my plan, he now has a lifestyle which incorporates healthy movements that he not only enjoys, but which challenge him as well.

Weight lost: 17.6lbs / 8kg
Exercise per week: 4–5 hours
Calories per day: 2,000
Reason for starting: I was overweight, unhappy with my body and my overall approach to food.

Have you tried losing weight before?
Yes. I've not been happy with the way I look for years, since uni. I did a 90-day plan online and I did get leaner, but I also got a bit skinny. The main problem was I got bored by the nutrition and the HIIT and launched myself off the wagon once it was done and soon the weight piled back on.

How did you feel when you started the plan?
Pretty unhappy, looking back – I was stagnating and eating my way into bad habits and a potentially unhealthy future. My weight, just after last Christmas, was shocking for what I usually am and something had to be done.

How do you feel now?
I feel amazing! I really enjoy being 'healthy'. I take pleasure in being able to jog a 5k at 8am along the river without getting a debilitating stitch. I love feeling stronger. I know that, when I eat dinner at night, I'm eating for what my body requires and not to excess. Seeing the side effects of that – losing weight, toning up – is even better.

What did you like the most in terms of following the plan?
I loved the progression in strength and the fact that the workouts were very

resistance-based. It gave a real sense of achievement once I started moving up the weights. I also loved the nutrition, being able to eat pasta, rice, bread, even chocolate! David's meals always delivered – enjoyable, easy to make and I never felt hungry. I think that's why this plan has been so successful for me – because the nutrition is enjoyable, which therefore makes it sustainable.

What exercises did you like the most or find gave you the most results?
The resistance training, and how progressive it is.

Was there anything you found tricky?
The workouts are quite long – not a bad thing in itself, but it meant I had to get up early to fit them in before work. But I just kept thinking of the end goal; you only get out what you put in!

Will you keep going with the plan now?
Without a shadow of a doubt. I'm in the best shape I've ever been in and I intend to build that to see what I can achieve. I'm taking care of myself now and that's a habit worth keeping. I can see this being a permanent lifestyle change. So thank you.

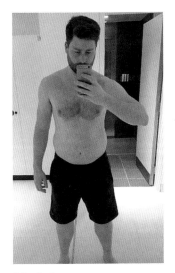
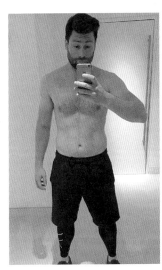

Week 1   Week 8

RESISTANCE TRAINING: HOME-BASED PLAN

If you can't – or don't want to – go to a gym, then this is the resistance plan for you. There are three sessions to choose from for the first four weeks, then three for the last four weeks of the plan, which are longer and more intense and so will ensure you are continuing to challenge your body and make progress.

If you find these exercises too hard, just get as far as you can for now. If you stick to the plan, you'll be able to do the full sets soon, I promise. If you find these exercises too easy, I recommend getting some dumbbells to add weight, increasing the number of reps, or trying out the Resistance Training: Gym-based Plan (page 227).

In this section, I've included photos of either myself or one of my clients, Alice, doing the exercises to help show you how to perform them correctly as you won't have a professional nearby to ask. Remember to start each session with a gentle five-minute warm up (see page 188). I recommend ending each session with at least five minutes of stretching as well (see page 186).

REPS, SETS, SUPERSETS AND CIRCUITS

The exercises will be shown with the number of repetitions (reps) and sets you need to perform. The instructions for each will look something like this:

Plank x 30 seconds
30-second rest
Superman x 8
30-second rest and repeat
Sets: 3

For this example above, you would hold the plank for 30 seconds, have a 30-second rest, do the Superman eight times, have a 30-second rest and then repeat this set another two times (so three rounds in total). The above is what is called a 'superset' because there is more than one exercise to complete. You will also find single 'sets' (only one exercise to complete), and 'circuits', with more than one exercise but less rest time between each one.

WEEKS 1–4: SESSION 1

Lunges x 10 each leg
30-second rest
Bench dips x 10
30-second rest and repeat
Sets: 4

LUNGES: Quads, hamstrings, glutes

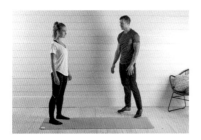 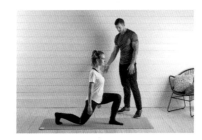 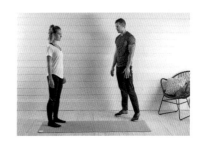

☐ Begin standing with your feet shoulder-width apart and your hands on your hips or by your sides.

☐ Step forward with one leg, flexing with the knees to drop your hips. Descend until your rear knee almost touches the floor. Your posture should remain upright, with your front knee staying above the front foot.

☐ Drive through the heel of the lead foot and extend both knees to raise yourself back up and return to your starting position. Repeat the lunge on the opposite side, repeating for the required number of reps on each leg.

BENCH DIPS: Abs, quads

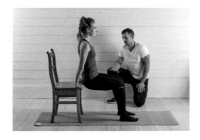 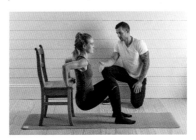 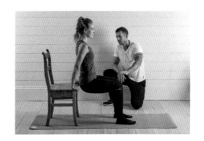

☐ Start by sitting at the edge of a bench or other stable surface, knees bent, feet flat on the floor. Place your hands on either side of your hips, palms down, fingers over the edge of the bench.

☐ Push gently up, straightening your arms, and shift your feet forward so your body is hanging just in front of the bench, with your knees bent to just over 90 degrees, and your feet flat on the floor. Keeping your back upright, bend your arms to slowly lower your hips by around 5–10cm, further if you find this too easy, briefly hold, then straighten your arms back to the starting position.

Squats x 12
30-second rest
Wall sit x 45-seconds
30-second rest
Glute kickbacks x 12 each leg
30-second rest
Star jumps x 45-seconds
30-second rest and repeat
Sets: 4

SQUATS: Quads, hamstrings, glutes

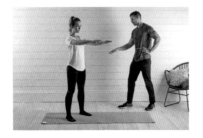 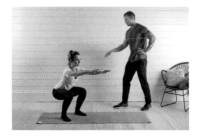 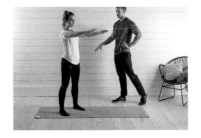

☐ Stand with your feet shoulder-width apart, with your hands behind your head or straight out in front of you.

☐ Bend your knees slightly and sit back with your hips. Continue down to full depth in a seated position if you're able to.

☐ Quickly reverse the motion until you return to the starting position. As you squat, make sure you're keeping your head and chest up while pushing your knees out.

WALL SIT: Quads, glutes, lower back, hamstings

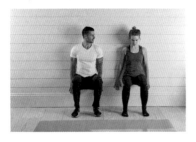

☐ Start with your back positioned against a wall, your feet slightly ahead of you.

☐ Slide your back downwards until you are in a squatting position. Your hips should be in line with your knees, and your shins at a 90-degree angle to your feet. Keep your arms and back firmly against the wall and hold for the required length of time.

GLUTE KICK-BACKS: Glutes, hamstrings

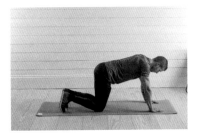 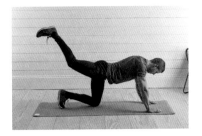 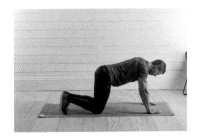

☐ Get on your hands and knees on the floor or an exercise mat with your arms straight and shoulder-width apart. Your head should be looking straight ahead or facing the floor and the bend of the knees should create a 90-degree angle between the hamstrings and the calves. This is your starting position.

☐ As you exhale, lift your right leg until the hamstrings are in line with your back, while maintaining the 90-degree-angle bend. Contract the glutes throughout this movement and hold the contraction at the top for a second. At the end of the movement your upper leg should be parallel to the floor while the calf should be perpendicular to it.

☐ Go back to the original position and repeat with the left leg. Continue the exercise using alternate legs, repeating the required number for each leg.

STAR JUMPS: Full body

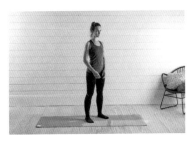 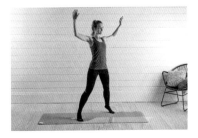 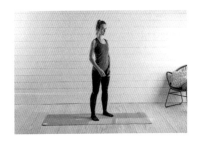

☐ Start with your feet shoulder-width apart with your arms by your sides.

☐ Start the movement by squatting down halfway and accelerating rapidly back up. Fully extend your whole body, spreading your legs and arms away from the body.

Plank x 30 seconds
30-second rest
Superman x 8
30-second rest and repeat
Sets: 3

PLANK: Abs, lower back, quads, hamstrings, glutes

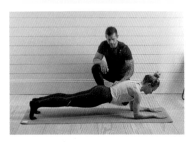

- ☐ Get into a push-up position on the floor but support the body with your forearms. Your arms should be bent at a 90-degree angle below your shoulders, and your weight balanced evenly between your forearms and your toes.

- ☐ Make sure your body is level and your core is engaged. Hold the position for the required length of time, ensuring you don't sag down or arch up.

- ☐ If you want to increase the difficulty, an arm or leg can be raised.

SUPERMAN: Lower back, glutes, hamstrings

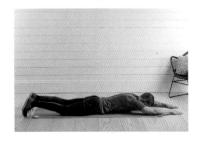 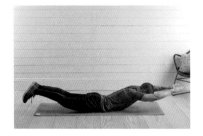 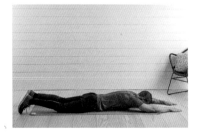

- ☐ Start by lying in a prone position on the floor (face down). Extend both arms fully in front of you. This is your starting position.

- ☐ Now raise both arms, legs, and chest off the floor simultaneously. Hold the movement at the top for 2 seconds then slowly lower back to your starting position. Focus on using the lower back and glutes for this exercise.

WEEKS 1–4: SESSION 2

Bulgarian split squats x 12 each side
30-second rest
Push-ups x 12
30-second rest and repeat
Sets: 4

BULGARIAN SPLIT SQUATS: Glutes and quads

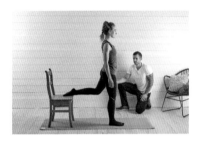 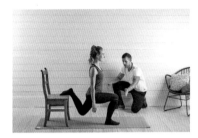 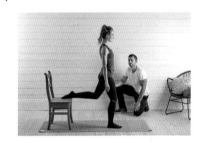

- ☐ Start in a staggered stance position with the rear foot elevated and resting on a bench or low chair, front foot forward. If you own them, hold a dumbbell in each hand down by your sides.

- ☐ Begin by lowering the body, flexing from the knee and hip. Maintain good posture throughout the movement. Keep the front knee in line/over the front foot as you perform the exercise.

- ☐ Drive through the heel at the bottom of the movement to extend the knee and hip and return to the starting position. Complete the required number of reps then switch sides and repeat on the other side.

PUSH-UPS: Pecs, triceps, shoulders, abs

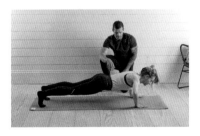 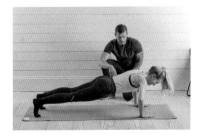 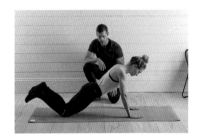

- ☐ Place your hands shoulder-width apart directly beneath your shoulders. Press down to raise your body, holding your torso up at arm's length, ensuring your weight evenly distributed between your hands and your toes.

- ☐ Next, lower yourself towards the ground until your chest is almost touching the floor, keeping your back and legs in line. From there, push upwards, returning to the original position while isolating the chest. If you find these too difficult then I suggest you can do the same movement from a kneeling position.

Squats x 12
30-second rest
Side plank raises x 12
30-second rest
Glute bridge x 12
30-second rest
Mountain climbers x 45-seconds
30-second rest and repeat
Sets: 4

SQUATS: Squats, hamstrings, glutes

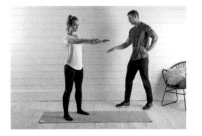 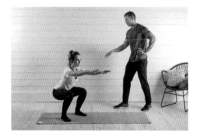 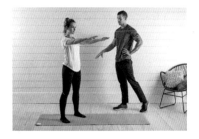

- ☐ Stand with your feet shoulder-width apart, with your hands behind your head or straight out in front of you.

- ☐ Bend your knees slightly and sit back with your hips. Continue down to full depth in a seated position if you're able to.

- ☐ Quickly reverse the motion until you return to the starting position. As you squat, make sure you're keeping your head and chest up while pushing your knees out.

SIDE PLANK RAISES: Obliques, lower back, glutes

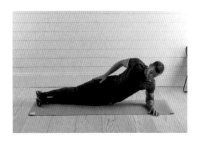 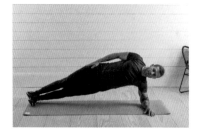 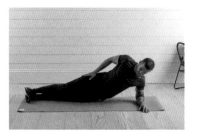

- ☐ Start by lying on your side on the floor with your feet together. Raise yourself up onto one elbow so it is directly below your shoulder.

- ☐ Raise your hips until your body is in a straight line from shoulder to feet while you contract your core muscles. Then lower your body down until your hip almost touches the ground. Raise your body back to the original side plank position. Repeat on both sides.

GLUTE BRIDGE: Glutes, abs, hamstrings, quads

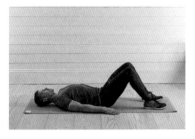 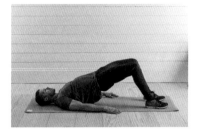 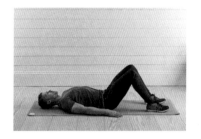

- ☐ Lie face up on the floor, with your knees bent and your feet flat on the ground. Keep your arms at the side of your body with your palms down.

- ☐ Lift your hips off the floor until your knees, hips and shoulders are forming a straight line. Squeeze the glutes hard and keep your abs tight so you don't overuse your back during the exercise.

- ☐ Hold the bridge position for a few seconds before lowering back down.

MOUNTAIN CLIMBERS: Full body, core

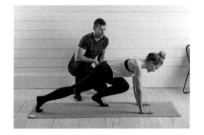 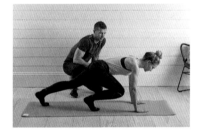 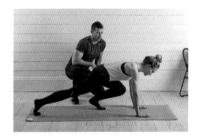

- ☐ Start in a push-up position, with your weight supported by your hands and toes. Bring one leg up until the knee is approximately under the hip. This will be your starting position.

- ☐ Explosively swap the position of your legs, extending the bent leg until it is straight and supported by the toe, and bringing the other knee in towards your chest. Repeat on alternating sides in a fast 'running' motion.

- ☐ Either repeat for the required number of reps or keep up at a high intensity for the required number of seconds.

Superman x 10
20-second rest
Bicycle x 10 each leg
20-second rest
Side plank x 20 seconds each side
20-second rest and repeat
Sets: 3

SUPERMAN: Lower back, glutes, hamstrings

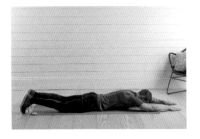 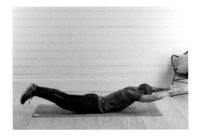 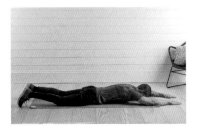

- [ ] Start by lying in a prone position on the floor (face down). Extend both arms fully in front of you. This is your starting position. Now raise both arms, legs, and chest off the floor simultaneously. Hold the movement at the top for 2 seconds then slowly lower back to your starting position. Focus on using the lower back and glutes for this exercise.

BICYCLE: Abs, quads

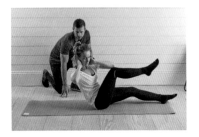 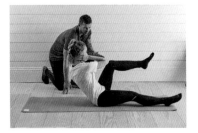 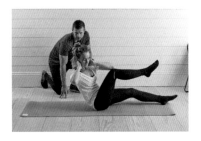

- [ ] Start by lying on your back on the floor with your hands behind your head, legs raised and knees pulled in towards your chest.
- [ ] Straighten one leg while pulling the other leg in at a 45-degree angle. As you do this, rotate your upper body, bringing the opposite elbow towards the leg that's coming in.
- [ ] Keep alternating sides rapidly in a cycling motion.

SIDE PLANK: Obliques, lower back, glutes

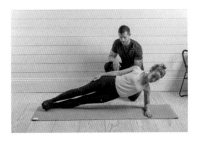 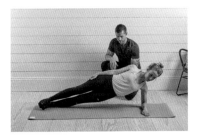 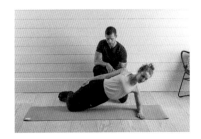

☐ Start by lying on your side on the floor with your feet together. Prop yourself up on one elbow, so your elbow is directly below your shoulder.

☐ Raise your hips until your body is in a straight line from shoulder to feet while you contract your core muscles. Hold your body in this raised position without lowering your hips for the allotted time. If you find this too hard, then you can rest on your lower leg. Do this by bending your legs at a 90 degree angle, as in image 3.

WEEKS 1–4: SESSION 3

Bench dips x 10
30-second rest
Skipping/Star jumps x 45-seconds
30-second rest and repeat

Reverse lunges x 10 each leg
30-second rest
Sets: 4

BENCH DIPS: Triceps, shoulders

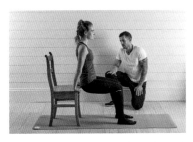 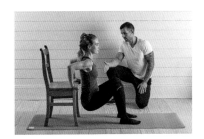 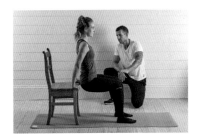

☐ Start by sitting at the edge of a bench or other stable surface, knees bent, feet flat on the floor. Place your hands on either side of your hips, palms down, fingers over the edge of the bench.

☐ Push gently up, straightening your arms, and shift your feet forward so your body is hanging just in front of the bench, with your knees bent to just over 90 degrees, and your feet flat on the floor. Keeping your back upright, bend your arms to slowly lower your hips by around 5–10cm, further if you find this too easy, briefly hold, then straighten your arms back to the starting position.

SKIPPING/STAR JUMPS: Full body

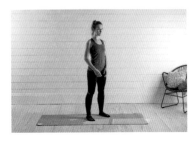 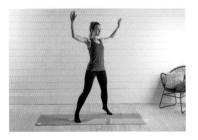 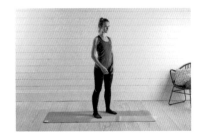

- ☐ Skipping: hold a skipping-rope handle in each hand. Keep your shoulders back with your elbows close to your sides. Bring the rope forward while rotating your wrists. Jump with both feet clearing the rope and the rope going overhead. Repeat the motion as quickly as you can.

- ☐ Star jumps: Start with your feet shoulder-width apart with your arms by your sides. Start the movement by squatting down halfway and accelerating rapidly back up. Fully extend your whole body, spreading your legs and arms away from the body.

REVERSE LUNGES: Quads, hamstrings, glutes

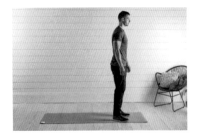 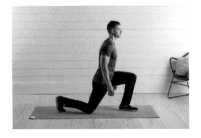 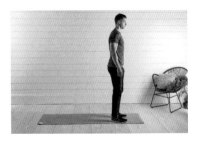

- ☐ Start in a standing position holding some dumbbells, if you have them, by your sides. Look forward, keeping your chest up, with your feet shoulder-width apart.

- ☐ Start the movement by taking a large step to the rear. Allow your knee and hip to flex so your body lowers. Descend until your knee almost touches the ground. Aim to keep the movement controlled and focus on proper posture. The knee should stay in line with the foot.

- ☐ Drive through the heel of the front leg to extend the knees and hips and return to the starting position. Alternate legs, doing the required number of reps on each leg.

Jogging high knees x 30 seconds
30-second rest
Walking plank x 8 each side
30-second rest
Squats x 12
30-second rest
Star jumps x 30
30-second rest and repeat
Sets: 4

JOGGING HIGH KNEES: Full body, legs

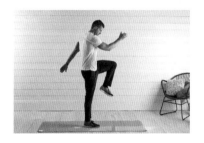 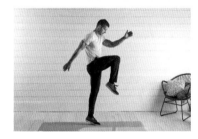 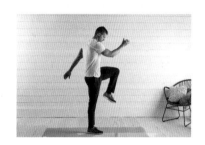

☐ Stand with your feet shoulder-width apart. Bend your arms at the elbow, so your hands are just above your hips, palms down.

☐ Jog on the spot with knees lifting up to make contact with your palms on every stride, keeping your back upright. Maintain the jog continuously for the required time before taking a rest.

WALKING PLANK: Abs, triceps, shoulders

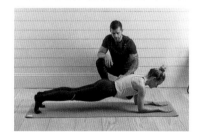 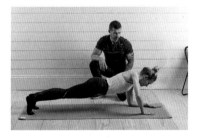 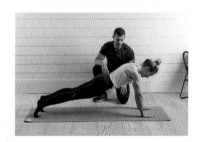

☐ Starting in a prone plank position, with your body in line resting on your forearms. One arm at a time, push from the original position into the elevated press-up position, keeping the core engaged with a flat back. Reverse this movement one arm at a time to the starting position. Repeat for the desired number of reps.

☐ If this movement is too challenging then you can start by performing it from your knees and progress up to your feet.

SQUATS: Quads, hamstrings, glutes

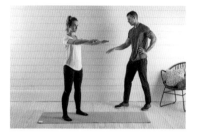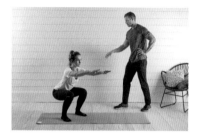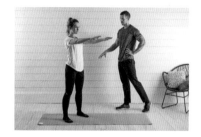

☐ Stand with your feet shoulder-width apart. You can place your hands behind your head. This is your starting position.

☐ Begin the movement by flexing at the hip, bending your knees slightly and sitting back with your hips. Continue down to full depth in a seated position if you're able to, then quickly reverse the motion until you return to the starting position. As you squat, make sure you're keeping your head and chest up while pushing your knees out.

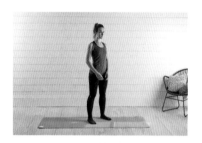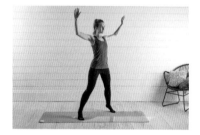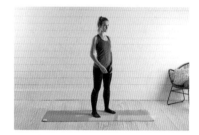

STAR JUMPS: Full body

☐ Start with your feet shoulder-width apart with your arms by your sides. Start the movement by squatting down halfway and accelerating rapidly back up.

☐ Fully extend your whole body, spreading your legs and arms away from the body.

Plank leg raises x 30-seconds per leg
30-second rest
Contralateral limb raises x 10 each side
30-second rest and repeat
Sets: 3

PLANK LEG RAISES: Abs, back, quads, hamstrings, glutes

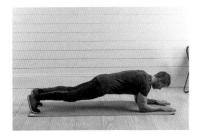 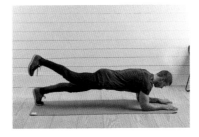 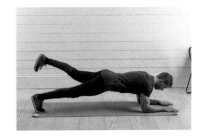

☐ Start in a push-up position with your hands under your shoulders. Your body should be in a straight line. Tightening your abs, lift one leg off the ground behind you until it reaches just above hip height. At the top position pause for a second before slowly returning to the starting position.

CONTRALATERAL LIMB RAISES: Back, glutes, quads, hamstrings

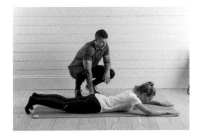 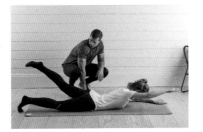 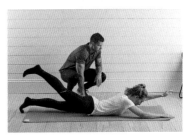

☐ Lie in a prone position (face down) on your stomach on the floor, with your toes pointed and your arms extended in front of you. Slowly raise one arm and the opposite leg a few inches off the ground. Alternate sides.

WEEKS 5–8: SESSION 1

Lunges x 12 each leg
Bench dips x 12
Mountain climbers x 45 seconds
45-second rest once all 3 are completed, then repeat
Sets: 5

LUNGES: Quads, hamstrings, glutes

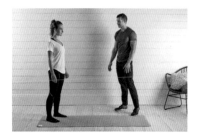 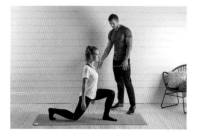 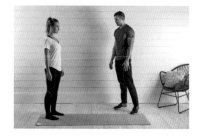

- ☐ Begin standing with your feet shoulder-width apart and your hands on your hips or by your sides.

- ☐ Step forward with one leg, flexing with the knees to drop your hips. Descend until your rear knee almost touches the floor. Your posture should remain upright, with your front knee staying above the front foot.

- ☐ Drive through the heel of the lead foot and extend both knees to raise yourself back up and return to your starting position. Repeat the lunge on the opposite side, repeating for the required number of reps on each leg.

BENCH DIPS: Triceps, shoulders

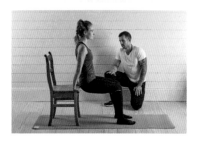 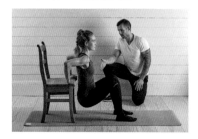 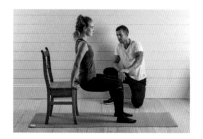

- ☐ Start by sitting at the edge of a bench or other stable surface, knees bent, feet flat on the floor. Place your hands on either side of your hips, palms down, fingers over the edge of the bench. Push gently up, straightening your arms, and shift your feet forward so your body is hanging just in front of the bench, with your knees bent to just over 90 degrees, and your feet flat on the floor.

- ☐ Keeping your back upright, bend your arms to slowly lower your hips by around 5–10cm, further if you find this too easy, briefly hold, then straighten your arms back to the starting position.

MOUNTAIN CLIMBERS: Full body, core

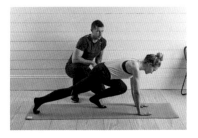 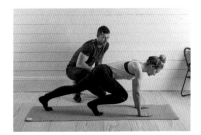 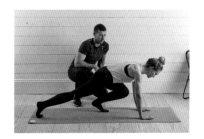

☐ Start in a push-up position, with your weight supported by your hands and toes. Bring one leg up until the knee is approximately under the hip. This will be your starting position.

☐ Explosively swap the position of your legs, extending the bent leg until it is straight and supported by the toe, and bringing the other knee in towards your chest. Repeat on alternating sides in a fast 'running' motion.

☐ Either repeat for the required number of reps or keep up at a high intensity for the required number of seconds.

Squats x 12
Single leg glute bridge x 12
Walk out push-ups x 10
Star jumps/Skipping x 60 seconds
45-second rest once all 4 are completed, then repeat
Sets: 5

SQUATS: Quads, hamstrings, glutes

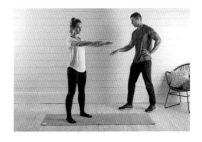 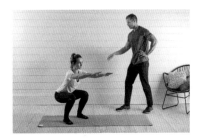 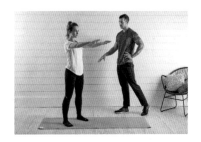

☐ Stand with your feet shoulder-width apart. You can place your hands behind your head. This is your starting position.

☐ Begin the movement by flexing at the hip, bending your knees slightly and sitting back with your hips. Continue down to full depth in a seated position if you're able to, then quickly reverse the motion until you return to the starting position. As you squat, make sure you're keeping your head and chest up while pushing your knees out.

SINGLE LEG GLUTE BRIDGE: Glutes, abs, hamstrings, quads

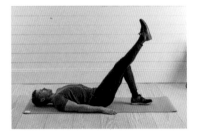 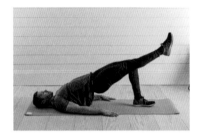 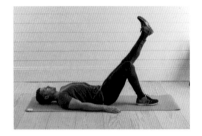

- ☐ Assume the glute bridge position, push your bum in the air, then lift and straighten one leg in line with the rest of your body, supporting your weight with the other leg.
- ☐ Hold the bridged position, then lower your leg. Repeat for the required number of reps then swap legs.

WALK OUT PUSH-UPS: Triceps, pecs, Shoulders, abs

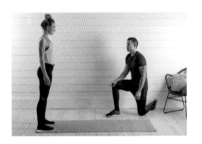 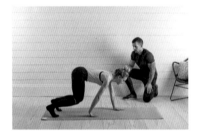 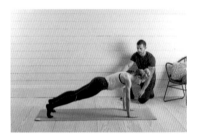

- ☐ Start in a standing position, feet hip-width apart. Bend at the hips then plant your hands on the floor, shoulder-width apart, a few inches ahead of your feet.
- ☐ Walk your hands forward until you're doing a push-up. Now reverse the entire movement and return to standing.

STAR JUMPS/SKIPPING: Full body

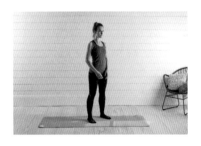 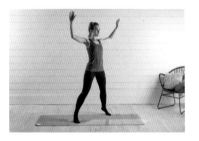 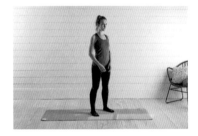

- ☐ Tips for star jumps: Start with your feet shoulder-width apart with your arms by your sides. Start the movement by squatting down halfway and accelerating rapidly back up, spreading your legs and arms away from the body.
- ☐ Tips for skipping: Keep your shoulders back with your elbows close to your sides . Repeat the motion with the skipping rope as quickly as you can.

Plank leg raises x 12 each side
Superman x 12
45-second rest once both exercises are completed, then and repeat
Sets: 4

PLANK LEG RAISES: Abs, back, quads, hamstrings, glutes

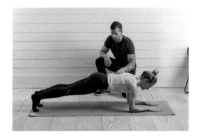 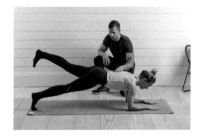 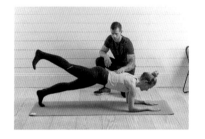

☐ Start in a push-up position with your hands under your shoulders. Your body should be in a straight line. Tightening your abs, lift one leg off the ground behind you until it reaches just above hip height. At the top position pause for a second before slowly returning to the starting position.

SUPERMAN: Lower back, glutes, hamstrings

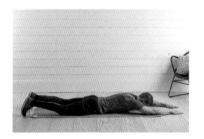 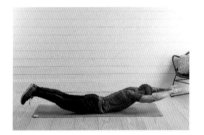 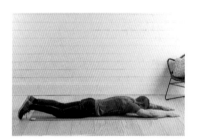

☐ Start by lying in a prone position on the floor (face down). Extend both arms fully in front of you. This is your starting position.

☐ Now raise both arms, legs, and chest off the floor simultaneously. Hold the movement at the top for 2 seconds then slowly lower back to your starting position. Focus on using the lower back and glutes for this exercise.

WEEKS 5–8: SESSION 2

Bulgarian split squats x 15 each side
Squats x 12
Push-ups x 12
Bench Dips x 12
60-second rest once all 4 are completed, then repeat
Sets: 5

BULGARIAN SPLIT SQUATS: Glutes, quads

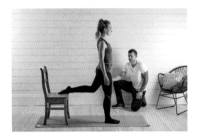 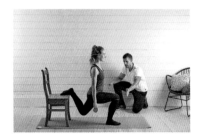 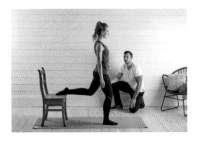

☐ Start in a staggered stance position with the rear foot elevated and resting on a bench or low chair, front foot forward. If you own them, hold a dumbbell in each hand down by your sides.

☐ Begin by lowering the body, flexing from the knee and hip. Maintain good posture throughout the movement. Keep the front knee in line/over the front foot as you perform the exercise.

☐ Drive through the heel at the bottom of the movement to extend the knee and hip and return to the starting position. Complete the required number of reps then switch sides and repeat on the other side.

SQUATS: Quads, hamstrings, glutes

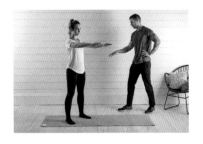 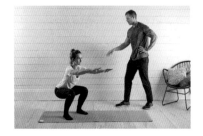 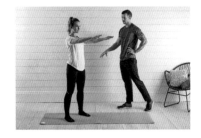

☐ Stand with your feet shoulder-width apart, with your hands behind your head or straight out in front of you.

☐ Bend your knees slightly and sit back with your hips. Continue down to full depth in a seated position if you're able to.

☐ Quickly reverse the motion until you return to the starting position. As you squat, make sure you're keeping your head and chest up while pushing your knees out.

PUSH-UPS: Pecs, triceps, shoulders, abs

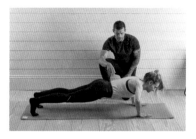 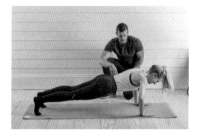 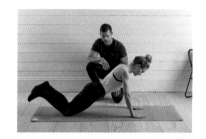

☐ Lie on the floor face down and place your hands shoulder-width apart directly beneath your shoulders. Press on your hands to raise your body, holding your torso up at arm's length and keeping your weight evenly distributed between your hands and your toes. Next, lower yourself towards the ground until your chest is almost touching the floor, keeping your back and legs in line. From there, push upwards, returning to the original position while isolating the chest.

☐ If you find these too difficult then I suggest you can do the same movement from a kneeling position.

BENCH DIPS: Triceps, shoulders

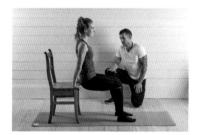 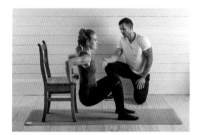 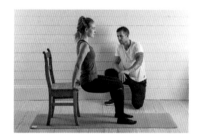

☐ Start by sitting at the edge of a bench or other stable surface, knees bent, feet flat on the floor. Place your hands on either side of your hips, palms down, fingers over the edge of the bench.

☐ Push gently up, straightening your arms, and shift your feet forward so your body is hanging just in front of the bench, with your knees bent to just over 90 degrees, and your feet flat on the floor. Keeping your back upright, bend your arms to slowly lower your hips by around 5-10cm, further if you find this too easy, briefly hold, then straighten your arms back to the starting position.

Lunges x 12 each side
Bicycle x 45sec
Single leg glute bridge x 10 each side
Mountain climber x 45 seconds
45-second rest once all 4 are completed, then repeat
Sets: 5

LUNGES: Quads, hamstrings, glutes

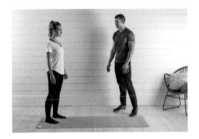 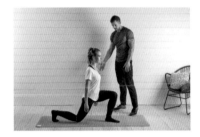 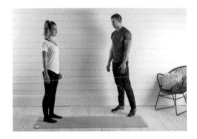

- ☐ Begin standing with your feet shoulder-width apart and your hands on your hips.

- ☐ Step forward with one leg, flexing with the knees to drop your hips. Descend until your rear knee almost touches the floor. Your posture should remain upright, with your front knee staying above the front foot.

- ☐ Drive through the heel of the lead foot and extend both knees to raise yourself back up and return to your starting position. Repeat the lunge on the opposite side, repeating for the required number of reps on each leg.

BICYCLE: Abs, quads

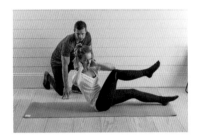 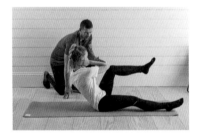 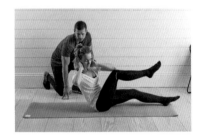

- ☐ Start by lying on your back on the floor with your hands behind your head, legs raised and knees pulled in towards your chest.

- ☐ Straighten one leg whilst pulling the other leg in at a 45-degree angle. As you do this, rotate your upper body, bringing the opposite elbow towards the leg that's coming in. Keep alternating sides rapidly in a cycling motion.

SINGLE LEG GLUTE BRIDGE: Glutes, abs, hamstrings, quads

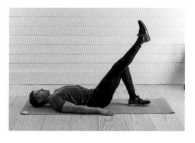 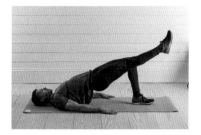 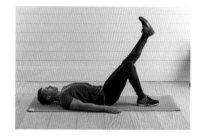

☐ Assume the glute bridge position (above) then lift and straighten one leg in line with the rest of your body, supporting your weight with the other leg.

☐ Hold the bridge position for a few seconds, then lower. Repeat for the required number of reps then swap legs.

MOUNTAIN CLIMBERS: Full body, core

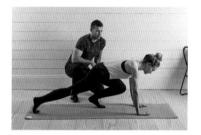 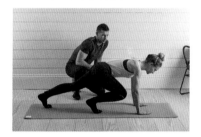 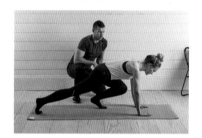

☐ Start in a push-up position, with your weight supported by your hands and toes. Bring one leg up until the knee is approximately under the hip. This will be your starting position.

☐ Explosively swap the position of your legs, extending the bent leg until it is straight and supported by the toe, and bringing the other knee in towards your chest. Repeat on alternating sides in a fast 'running' motion.

☐ Either repeat for the required number of reps or keep up at a high intensity for the required number of seconds.

Side plank raises x 12 each side
Plank x 45 seconds
Contralaterel limb raises x 12 each side

45-second rest once all 3 are completed,
then repeat
Sets: 4

SIDE PLANK RAISES: Obliques, lower back, glutes

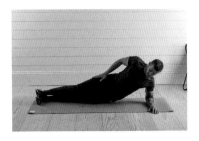 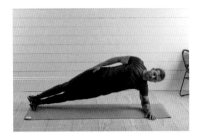 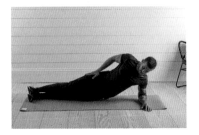

☐ Start by lying on your side on the floor with your feet together. Raise yourself up onto one elbow so it is directly below your shoulder.

☐ Raise your hips until your body is in a straight line from shoulder to feet while you contract your core muscles. Then lower your body down until your hip almost touches the ground. Raise your body back to the original side plank position. Repeat on both sides.

PLANK: Abs, lower back, quads, hamstrings, glutes

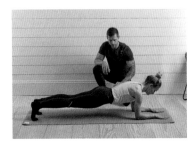

☐ Get into a push-up position on the floor but support the body with your forearms. Your arms should be bent at a 90-degree angle below your shoulders, and your weight balanced evenly between your forearms and your toes.

☐ Make sure your body is level and your core is engaged. Hold the position for the required length of time, ensuring you don't sag down or arch up.

☐ If you want to increase the difficulty, an arm or leg can be raised.

CONTRALATERAL LIMB RAISES: Back, glutes, quads, hamstrings

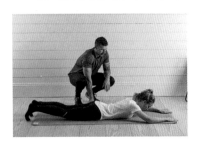 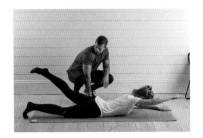 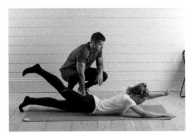

☐ Lie in a prone position (face down) on your stomach on the floor, with your toes pointed and your arms extended in front of you. Slowly raise one arm and the opposite leg a few inches off the ground. Alternate sides.

WEEKS 5–8: SESSION 3

Step-ups x 10 each leg
Reverse lunges x 10 each leg
Bench dips x 10
Burpees x 12

60-second rest once all 4 are completed,
then repeat
Sets: 5

STEP-UPS: Quads, hamstrings, glutes

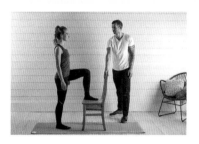 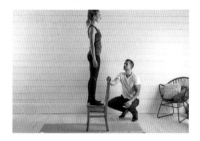 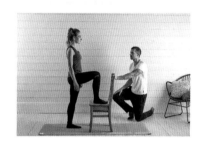

☐ Stand in front of a step or low bench. Step up one foot at a time then repeat with the opposite foot, alternating between legs.

REVERSE LUNGES: Quads, hamstrings, glutes

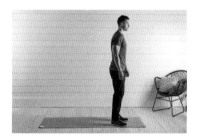 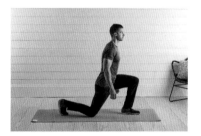 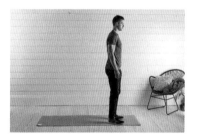

☐ Start in a standing position holding some dumbbells, if you have them. Look forward, keeping your chest up, with your feet shoulder-width apart. Take a large step to the rear. Allow your knee and hip to flex so your body lowers.

☐ Descend until your knee almost touches the ground. Aim to keep the movement controlled and focus on proper posture. The knee should stay in line with the foot. Drive through the heel of the front leg to extend the knees and hips and return to the starting position. Alternate legs, doing the required number of reps on each leg.

BENCH DIPS: Triceps, shoulders

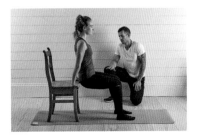 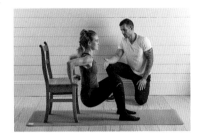 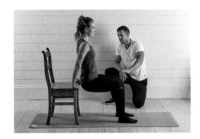

☐ Start by sitting at the edge of a bench or other stable surface, knees bent, feet flat on the floor. Place your hands on either side of your hips, palms down, fingers over the edge of the bench.

☐ Push gently up, straightening your arms, and shift your feet forward so your body is hanging just in front of the bench, with your knees bent to just over 90 degrees, and your feet flat on the floor. Keeping your back upright, bend your arms to slowly lower your hips by around 5–10cm, further if you find this too easy, briefly hold, then straighten your arms back to the starting position.

BURPEES: Full body

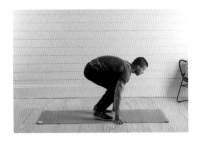 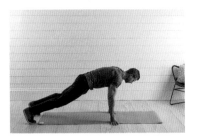 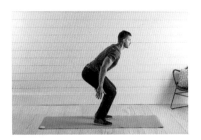

☐ Start in a squat position with feet hip-width apart and your hands on the floor in front of you. Now jump your feet backwards into a push-up position, then jump straight back into the squat position.

☐ Finish by leaping as high as possible, landing back on your feet and dropping back into a squat.

Squats jumps x 15
Walking plank x 10 each side
Push-ups x 12
Star jumps x 60 seconds
45-second rest once all 4 are completed, then repeat
Sets: 5

SQUAT JUMP: Quads, hamstrings, glutes, calves

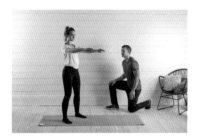 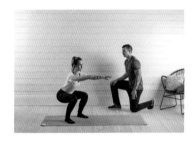 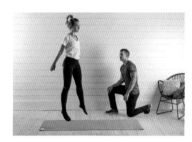

☐ Start by standing with your feet shoulder-width apart. Begin moving into a regular squat position while engaging your core, then explosively jump upwards. Land as softly as possible and immediately return back to a squat position.

WALKING PLANK: Abs, triceps, shoulders

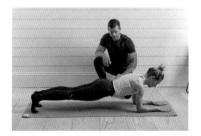 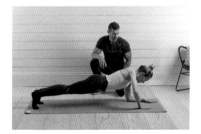 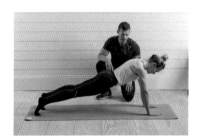

☐ Starting in a prone plank position, with your body in line resting on your forearms. One arm at a time, push from the original position into the elevated press-up position, keeping the core engaged with a flat back. Reverse this movement one arm at a time to the starting position. Repeat for the desired number of reps.

☐ If this movement is too challenging then you can start by performing it from your knees and progress up to your feet.

PUSH-UPS: Pecs, triceps, shoulders, abs

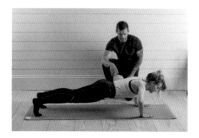 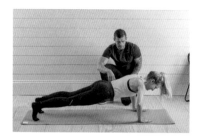 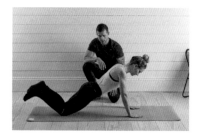

- ☐ Lie on the floor face down and place your hands shoulder-width apart directly beneath your shoulders. Press on your hands to raise your body, holding your torso up at arm's length and keeping your weight evenly distributed between your hands and your toes. Next, lower yourself towards the ground until your chest is almost touching the floor, keeping your back and legs in line. From there, push upwards, returning to the original position while isolating the chest.

- ☐ If you find these too difficult then I suggest you can do the same movement from a kneeling position.

STAR JUMPS: Full body

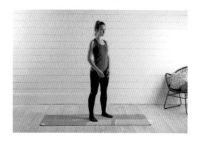 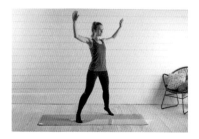 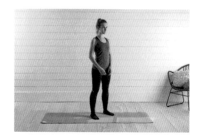

- ☐ Start with your feet shoulder-width apart with your arms by your sides.

- ☐ Start the movement by squatting down halfway and accelerating rapidly back up. Fully extend your whole body, spreading your legs and arms away from the body.

Glute kick-back x 12 each side
Contralateral limb raises x 10 each side
Skipping/Star jumps x 60 seconds
45-second rest once all 3 are completed, then repeat
Sets: 4

GLUTE KICK-BACKS: Glutes, hamstrings

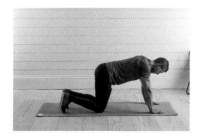 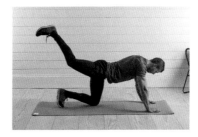 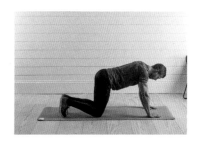

☐ Get on your hands and knees on the floor or an exercise mat with your arms straight and shoulder-width apart. Your head should be looking straight ahead or down at the floor and the bend of the knees should create a 90-degree angle between the hamstrings and the calves. This is your starting position.

☐ As you exhale, lift your right leg until the hamstrings are in line with your back, while maintaining the 90-degree-angle bend. Contract the glutes throughout this movement and hold the contraction at the top for a second. At the end of the movement the upper leg should be parallel to the floor while the calf should be perpendicular to it.

☐ Go back to the original position and repeat with the left leg. Continue the exercise using alternate legs, repeating the required number for each leg.

CONTRALATERAL LIMB RAISES: Back, glutes, quads, hamstrings

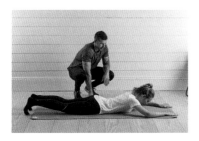 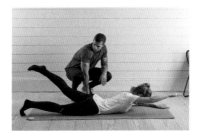 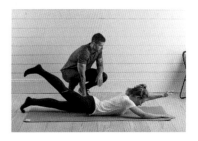

☐ Lie in a prone position (face down) on your stomach on the floor, with your toes pointed and your arms extended in front of you. Slowly raise one arm and the opposite leg a few inches off the ground. Alternate sides.

SKIPPING/STAR JUMPS: Full body

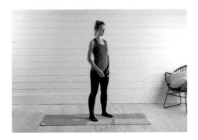 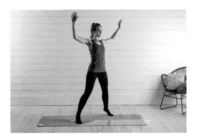 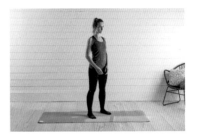

☐ Tips for star jumps: Start with your feet shoulder-width apart with your arms by your sides. Start the movement by squatting down halfway and accelerating rapidly back up, spreading your legs and arms away from the body.

☐ Tips for skipping: Keep your shoulders back with your elbows close to your sides. Repeat the motion with the skipping rope as quickly as you can.

RESISTANCE TRAINING: GYM-BASED PLAN

On the next few pages, you'll find three levels of exercise plan with progressing difficulty. Within each level are three sessions to complete each week if time allows. If you don't have time to perform all three sessions each week then select either one or two depending on time and do these consistently each week. If you haven't done any of the home-based exercises, then see page 198 for an explanation of how the instructions for each exercise works. N.B. you will see the supersets in this plan are labelled as 1a,1b; 2a, 2b, 2c etc. This means they should be performed as a pair/group alternately, separated by a rest if instructed.

Unlike the home-based plan, there are male and female plans here as some weight-related exercises are better suited to men and some for women when trying to achieve a fitter and leaner physique. (But the exercises are by no means easier in one plan or the other!) As with the home-based exercises, you should start each session with a gentle five-minute warm up (see page 188). I recommend ending each session with at least five minutes of stretching (page 186).

A note about weights: as I said on page 193, always use the heaviest weight you can lift safely and sustainably throughout your session. If you are working with the correct intensity, you'll probably find it tricky to do the same number again and again each set, as your muscles will get tired. If that's the case, try reducing the number of reps on the subsequent sets, rather than reducing the weight you're using. So, for example, if you're doing 4x12 bench press, then you can do 12 reps, followed by 11 reps, then 10, then 9. If you do this, keep a note of the exact weight you're lifting and use it week after week until you can perform the full 4x12 rep sets. Once you've achieved this, increase the weight and repeat.

If you would like to see photos of how to use the equipment, you can find pictures on my website: www.davidkingsbury.co.uk/movements. Descriptions of all the exercises and how to do them are on pages 240–249 – I would recommend reading them through thoroughly first, giving them a practice run so that you're confident you know what you're doing, and then doing the session. Before long it will be second nature.

LEVEL 1 – FEMALE

SESSION 1

1a Dumbbell shoulder press (page 244) x 12

60-second rest

1b Single arm rows (page 248) x 12 each arm

60-second rest and repeat

Sets: 4

2a Squats (Home-based exercises, page 200) x 12

60-second rest

2b Glute bridge (Home-based exercises, page 205) x 12

60-second rest and repeat

Sets: 4

BODYWEIGHT CIRCUIT:

Lunges (Home-based exercises, page 199) x 12 each side

Dumbbell curl and press (page 242) x 12

Glute kick-backs (Home-based exercises, page 201) x 12 each side

Bench dips (page 199) x 12

2-minute rest once all 4 are completed, then repeat

Sets: 4

SESSION 2

1a Dumbbell front squat (page 243) x 12

60-second rest

1b Lunges (Home-based exercises page 199) x 12 each leg

60-second rest and repeat

Sets: 4

2 Dumbbell clean and press (page 242) x 15

30-second rest and repeat

Sets: 4

3a Leg press, single leg (page 246) x 12 each side

30-second rest

3b Plank (Home-based exercises, page 202) x 30-seconds

30-second rest

3c Squats (Home-based exercises, page 200) x 12

30-second rest and repeat

Sets: 3

Cycle or rowing machine (your choice)

20 seconds very high intensity; 10 seconds low intensity

Sets: 8 (total time: 4 minutes)

(This is known as a Tabata session. See page 252 for more details.)

SESSION 3

1a Dumbbell thruster (page 244) x 12

60-second rest

1b Lat pull down (page 246) x 12

60-second rest and repeat

Sets: 4

2a Cable punch (page 241) x 12 each arm

60-second rest

2b Single arm rows (page 248) x 12 each arm

60-second rest and repeat

Sets: 4

BODYWEIGHT CIRCUIT:

Reverse lunges (Home-based exercises, page 208) x 12 each side

Walking plank (Home-based exercisess, page 209) x 12

Squats (Home-based exercisese, page 200) x 12

Mountain climbers (Home-based exercises, page 205) x 12 each side

2-minute rest once all 4 are completed, then repeat

Sets: 3

LEVEL 2 – FEMALE

SESSION 1

1a Dumbbell front squat (page 243) x 10

1b Dumbbell reverse lunges (page 243) x 10 each leg

60-second rest once both are completed, then repeat

Sets: 5

2a Dumbbell curl and press (page 242) x 12

2b Single arm rows (page 248) x 12 each side

60-second rest once both are completed, then repeat

Sets: 5

BODYWEIGHT CIRCUIT:

Glute kick-backs (Home-based exercises, page 201) x 12 each side

Push-ups (Home-based exercises, page 203) x 8

Bench dips (Home-based exercises, page 199) x 8

Lateral raises (page 246) x 12

Contralateral limb raises (Home-based exercises, page 211) x 12

90-second rest once all 5 are completed, then repeat

Sets: 5

SESSION 2

1 Bulgarian split squat (Home-based exercises, page 203) x 12 each side

60-second rest and repeat

Sets: 4

2 Lunges (Home-based exercises, page 199) x 12 each side

60-second rest and repeat

Sets: 4

3a Leg press (page 246) x 12

60-second rest

3b Dumbbell clean and press (page 242) x 12

60-second rest and repeat

Sets: 5

DUMBELL CIRCUIT:

Dumbbell shoulder press (page 244) x 12

Dumbbell bent over row (page 241) x 12

Dumbbell reverse lunges (page 243) x 12

Dumbbell front squats (page 243) x 12

2-minute rest once all 4 are completed, then repeat

Sets: 4

SESSION 3

1a Dumbbell shoulder press (page 244) x 10

60-second rest

1b Lat pull down (page 246) x 10

60-second rest and repeat

Sets: 5

2a Lunge and shoulder press (page 246) x 12

2b Renegade row (page 248) x 12 each side

2c Single leg glute bridge (Home-based exercises, page 214) x 12 each

leg

90-second rest once all 3 are completed, then repeat

Sets: 5

COMBO INTERVALS:

Rowing machine x 60-seconds at sprint pace

Burpees (Home-based exercises, page 222) x 12

Squats (Home-based exercises, page 200) x 12

2-minute rest once all 3 are completed, then repeat

Sets: 4

LEVEL 3 – FEMALE

SESSION 1

1a Dumbbell thruster (page 244) x 10
1b Dumbbell step-ups (page 244) x 10
40-second rest and repeat
Sets: 5

2a Pivot barbell shoulder press (page 247) x 12 each arm
2b Pivot barbell single arm row (page 247) x 12 each arm
60-second rest and repeat
Sets: 5

BODYWEIGHT CIRCUIT:
Glute kick-back (Home-based exercises, page 201) x 12 each side
Push-ups (Home-based exercises, page 203) x 8
Bench dips (Home-based exercises, page 199) x 8
Lateral raises (page 246) x 12
Rear delt raises (page 248) x 12
90-second rest once all 5 are completed, then repeat
Sets: 5

SESSION 2

1 Barbell back squat (page 240) x 10
60-second rest and repeat
Sets: 5

2 Barbell glute bridge (page 240) x 12
60-second rest and repeat
Sets: 4

3a Leg press, single leg (page 246) x 12 each leg

60-second rest

3b Dumbbell clean and press (page 242) x 12

60-second rest and repeat

Sets: 5

KETTLEBELL CIRCUIT:

Kettlebell single arm clean and press (page 245) x 10 each side

Kettlebell goblet squat (page 245) x 10

Kettlebell swing (page 245) x 10

Kettlebell deadlift (page 245) x 10

2-minute rest once all 4 are completed, then repeat

Sets: 4

SESSION 3

1a Dumbbell shoulder press (page 244) x 8

60-second rest

1b Pull-up (page 248) x 8

60-second rest and repeat

Sets: 5

2a Swiss ball hamstring curl (page 249) x 12

2b Swiss ball atomic push-up (page 249) x 12

2c Swiss ball roll-out (page 249) x 8

90-second rest once all 3 are completed, then repeat

Sets: 5

COMBO INTERVALS:

Rowing machine x 60 seconds at sprint pace

Squat jumps (Home-based exercises, page 223) x 12

Reverse lunges (Home-based exercises, page 208) x 12 each side

2-minute rest once all 3 are completed, then repeat

Sets: 5

LEVEL 1 – MALE

SESSION 1

1a Dumbbell bench press (page 241) x 12

60-second rest

1b Single arm rows (page 248) x 12 each arm

60-second rest and repeat

Sets: 4

2a Dumbbell shoulder press (page 244) x 12

60-second rest

2b Rear delt raise (page 248) x 12

60-second rest and repeat

Sets: 4

BODYWEIGHT CIRCUIT:

Push-ups (Home-based exercises, page 203) x 12

Reverse lunges (Home-based exercises, page 208) x 12 each leg

Glute bridge (Home-based exercises, page 205) x 12

Squats (Home-based exercises, page 200) x 12

Bench dips (Home-based exercises, page 199) x 12

2-minute rest once all 5 are completed, then repeat

Sets: 3

SESSION 2

1a Dumbbell front squat (page 243) x 12

60-second rest

1b Lunges (Home-based exercises, page 199) x 12 each leg

60-second rest and repeat

Sets: 4

2 Glute bridge (Home-based exercises, page 205) x 12

60-second rest and repeat

Sets: 4

3a Leg press, single leg (page 246) x 12 each leg

30-second rest

3b Plank (Home-based exercises, page 202) x 30-seconds

30-second rest

3c Dumbbell calf raises (page 242) x 30

30-second rest and repeat

Sets: 3

Cycle or rowing machine (your choice)

20 seconds very high intensity; 10 seconds low intensity

Sets: 8 (total time: 4 minutes)

(This is known as a Tabata session. See page 252 for more details.)

SESSION 3

1a Dumbbell incline bench press (page 243) x 12

60-second rest

1b Lat pull down (page 246) x 12

60-second rest and repeat

Sets: 4

2a Dumbbell bench press (page 241) x 12

60-second rest

2b Single arm rows (page 248) x 12 each arm

60-second rest and repeat

Sets: 4

BODYWEIGHT CIRCUIT:

Walking plank (Home-based exercises, page 209) x 12

Reverse lunges (Home-based exercises, page 208) x 12 each leg

Bench dips (Home-based exercises, page 199) x 12

Squats (Home-based exercises, page 200) x 12

Mountain climbers (Home-based exercises, page 205) x 12 each side

2-minute rest once all 5 are completed, then repeat

Sets: 3

LEVEL 2 – MALE

SESSION 1

1a Barbell incline bench press (page 240) x 10

60-second rest

1b Dumbbell bent over row (page 241) x 10

60-second rest and repeat

Sets: 5

2a Dumbbell bench press (page 241) x 12

60-second rest

2b Single arm rows (page 248) x 12 each arm

60-second rest and repeat

Sets: 5

3a Tricep push-down (page 249) x 12

3b Push-ups (Home-based exercises, page 203) x 12

3c Dumbbell curls (page 242) x 12

90-second rest once all 3 are completed, then repeat

Sets: 4

4a Hammer curls (page 244) x 12

4b Lateral raises (page 246) x 12

4c Rear delt raises (page 248) x 12

90-second rest once all 3 are completed, then repeat

Sets: 4

SESSION 2

1 Bulgarian split squat (see Home-based exercises, page 203) x 10 each side

60-second rest

Sets: 5

2 Reverse lunges (Home-based exercises, page 208) x 12 each side

60-second rest and repeat

Sets: 4

3a Leg press (page 246) x 12

60-second rest

3b Dumbbell clean and press (page 242) x 12

60-second rest and repeat

Sets: 5

DUMBELL CIRCUIT:

Dumbbell shoulder press (page 244) x 12

Dumbbell bent over row (page 241) x 12

Dumbbell dead lift (page 243) x 12

Dumbbell reverse lunges (page 243) x 12 each leg

Dumbbell front squats (page 243) x 12

2-minute rest once all 5 are completed, then repeat

Sets: 4

SESSION 3

1a Dumbbell shoulder press (page 244) x 10

60-second rest

1b Lat pull down (page 246) x 10

60-second rest and repeat

Sets: 5

2a Dumbbell clean and press (page 242) x 12

30-second rest

2b Renegade row (page 248) x 12 each side

2c Push-ups (Home-based exercises, page 203) x 12

90-second rest and repeat

Sets: 5

COMBO INTERVALS:

Rowing machine x 60-seconds at sprint pace

Burpees (Home-based exercises, page 222) x 12

Squats (Home-based exercises, page 200) x 12

2-minute rest once all 3 are completed, then repeat

Sets: 5

LEVEL 3 – MALE

SESSION 1

In these exercises, you will be doing what is known as drop sets. This means you perform the exercise for the required number of reps, then drop the weight to enable you to do the remaining reps, although don't worry if you're struggling.

1 Barbell bench press (page 240) x 8+8 drop set

90-second rest and repeat

Sets: 5

2 Dumbell bent over row (page 241) x 8+8 drop set

90-second rest and repeat

Sets: 5

3a Dumbbell incline bench press (page 243) x 12

30-second rest

3b Single arm rows (page 248) x 12 each arm

60-second rest and repeat

Sets: 5

3a Tricep dips (page 249) x 10

3b Push-ups (Home-based exercises, page 203) x 10

3c Bench dips (Home-based exercises, page 199) x 10

30-second rest

3d Dumbbell incline curls (page 243) x 12+12 drop set

60-second rest and repeat

Sets: 5

SESSION 2

1 Bulgarian split squat (Home-based exercises, page 203) x 8 each leg

60-second rest and repeat

Sets: 5

2 Dumbbell front squats (page 243) x 8

60-second rest and repeat

Sets: 4

3a Lunges (Home-based exercises, page 212) x 12 each leg

60-second rest

3b Barbell glute bridge (page 240) x 10

60-second rest and repeat

Sets: 5

COMBO INTERVALS:

Rowing machine x 60 seconds at sprint pace

Step-ups (Home-based exercises, page 221) x 12 each side

Mountain climbers (Home-based exercises, page 219) x 12 each side

2-minute rest once all 3 completed, then repeat

Sets: 5

SESSION 3

1a Pull-ups (page 248) x 8

60-second rest

1b Dumbbell incline bench press (page 243) x 8

60-second rest and repeat

Sets: 5

2a Dumbbell bench press (page 241) x 12

2b Push-ups (Home-based exercises, page 203) x 12

2c Seated row (page 248) x 20

60-second rest once all 3 completed, then repeat

Sets: 5

3a Tricep dips (page 249) x 12

15-second rest

3b Negative pull-up (page 247) x 30-seconds

3c Dumbbell curls (page 242) x 12

90-second rest and repeat

Sets: 4

4a Burpees (Home-based exercises, page 222) x 12

4b Squats (Home-based exercises, page 200) x 12

60-second rest and repeat

Sets: 4

THE EXERCISES

For further information, instruction and support on these exercises, you can visit my website at www.davidkingsbury.co.uk/movements

BARBELL BACK SQUAT: Quads, hamstrings, glutes

- ☐ Start with a barbell held in your hands, palms forward, supported on top of the traps. Keep the chest up and the head facing forward. Stand with a hip-width stance with the feet turned out as needed.
- ☐ Lower your body into a squat, flexing the knees and hips. Keep the torso as upright as possible. Continue all the way down until your thighs are just passed parallel to the ground, keeping the weight on the front of the heel. At the bottom of the movement, reverse the motion, driving the weight upward.

BARBELL BENCH PRESS: Pecs, triceps, shoulders

- ☐ Load the bar to an appropriate weight in the rack. Lying flat on a press bench, grab the barbell with an overhand grip, hands shoulder-width apart, and hold it above your chest. You should feel a slight arch in the back. Extend the arms upward, locking out elbows. This is the starting position.
- ☐ Lower the bar straight down in a controlled, slow movement to the top of your chest.

Pause, then press the bar in a straight line back up to the starting position.

BARBELL GLUTE BRIDGE: Glutes, abs, hamstrings, quads

- ☐ Start seated on the ground with a loaded barbell over your legs. Using a pad or towel on the bar will reduce the discomfort caused by the pressure of the bar. Roll the bar so that it is directly above your hips, and lay down flat on the floor. Hold the barbell in your hands, palms downwards, with straight arms.
- ☐ Drive through the heels, extending your hips vertically. Your weight will be supported by your upper back and your heels.
- ☐ Lift up as far as possible, then reverse the motion to return to the starting position.

BARBELL INCLINE BENCH PRESS: Pecs, triceps, shoulders

- ☐ Load the bar to an appropriate weight in the rack. Lying in the incline position, grab the barbell with an overhand grip, hands shoulder-width apart, and hold it above your chest. You should feel a slight arch in the back. Extend the arms upward, locking out elbows. This is the starting position.

Lower the bar straight down in a controlled, slow movement to the top of your chest. Pause, then press the bar in a straight line back up to the starting position.

CABLE PUNCH: Triceps, pecs, shoulders

☐ Set a cable machine pulley to chest height then attach a single handle. Grab the handle with your right hand with your back to the machine. Stagger your feet, with your left foot in front. Hold the handle outside your shoulder with your hand at the same height as your shoulder.

☐ Start the movement with your left arm straight out in front of you. Push the handle forward and straighten your right arm out in front of you. As you push the handle forward, bring your left arm back. Complete the designated number of reps on both sides.

CABLE SINGLE ARM ROW: Lats, middle and upper back, biceps

☐ Set a cable machine pulley to elbow height then attach a single handle. Grab the handle with your right hand with your front to the machine. Stagger your feet, with your left foot in front. Hold the handle extended in front of you.

☐ Start the movement with your right arm straight out in front of you and your left arm at your side. Pull the handle towards your body until your hand is in line with your body. As you pull the handle towards you, push your left arm out. Complete the designated number of reps on both sides.

DUMBBELL BENCH PRESS: Triceps, pecs

☐ Begin lying on a press bench, with your legs hanging off the end, knees bent, feet on the floor, one dumbbell in each hand. Hold your arms straight out above you, dumbbells almost but not quite touching.

☐ Slowly lower the dumbbells outwards, bending at the elbow, keeping your forearms vertical, until the dumbbells are level with your head. Pause for a moment then lift the dumbbells back up. Repeat until you have completed your reps.

DUMBBELL BENT OVER ROW: Lats, middle and upper back, biceps

☐ Start standing up, feet hip-width apart, with a dumbbell in each hand and your palms facing your torso. Bring your torso forward by bending at the waist and bend your knees slightly. Make sure to keep your back straight until it is almost parallel to the floor. The weights should be positioned hanging directly in front of you as your arms hang perpendicular to the floor and your torso.

☐ Lift the dumbbells to your side while keeping the back position fixed. Keep your elbows close to the body. At the top position, squeeze the back muscles. Lower the weights slowly again to the starting position.

DUMBBELL BULGARIAN SPLIT SQUATS: Biceps, glutes, quads

☐ See bodyweight exercise instructions (page 203), but hold a dumbbell in each hand.

DUMBBELL CALF RAISES: Biceps, calfs

☐ With a dumbbell in each hand and with arms straight at your sides, rest the ball of each foot on a weight plate or low step.

☐ Keep your body upright with your heels resting firmly on the floor.

☐ Push through the balls of your feet into the plate/step, rising up as high as possible on your toes. Pause, then lower back to starting position.

DUMBBELL CLEAN AND PRESS: Full body, deltoids

☐ Start in a standing position with a dumbbell in both hands, legs hip-width apart. Your palms should be facing your body and your arms hanging at your side.

☐ Lower the weights downwards by flexing your knees and hips, so you are in a low squat with your weights almost touching the floor at either side of you. This is your starting position.

☐ The movement is initiated explosively by extending the hips, knees and ankles to accelerate the weights upward. At the same time raise the weights above your head until you are in a standing position with your arms straight up in a full press overhead.

☐ After full extension, return to a squat position. Allow the arms to bend, guiding the dumbbells first to your shoulders then back to your sides on your way down.

DUMBBELL CURL: Biceps

☐ Begin standing with your feet shoulder-width apart, a dumbbell in each hand, arms hanging down, palms facing forward.

☐ Without using your back muscles, bend your arms at the elbow to bring the dumbbells towards your head. Finish with your palms facing towards you. Do not let the dumbbells touch each other. Hold for a moment, then lower slowly back to the starting position.

DUMBBELL CURL AND PRESS: Biceps, shoulders

☐ Start in a standing position with a dumbbell in each hand. Arms should be by your sides with your palms facing forward. Look ahead, with your chest up and your feet shoulder-width apart.

☐ Start by flexing the elbows to curl the weight up to shoulder height. Do not rely on momentum or use the shoulders.

☐ Once the weights are at the top, start the pressing movement by extending the arm and flexing the shoulder while rotating the weights. They should end in a neutral position above the head, palms facing each other.

☐ Pause and, in a controlled manner, reverse the movement to return to the starting position.

DUMBBELL DEADLIFT: Lower back, hamstrings, glutes, quadriceps

☐ Lift a couple of dumbbells and hold them by your sides at arm's length. Stand with your torso straight and your legs spaced at a shoulder-width apart. The knees should be slightly bent. Keeping the knees stationary, lower the dumbbells over the top of your feet by bending at the waist while keeping your back straight. Keep moving down until you feel your hamstrings stretch. It is a similar motion to picking something up from the floor.

☐ Start bringing your torso up straight again by extending your hips and waist until you are back to the starting position.

DUMBBELL FRONT SQUAT: Quads, hamstrings, glutes

☐ Standing with your feet shoulder-width apart, a dumbbell in each hand, bring the dumbbells to shoulder height, so that one end of each dumbbell rests on top of each shoulder with your elbows facing forward. This is your starting position.

☐ Lower your body until your thighs are parallel to the ground, making sure the

weight stays in your heels. Keep your face forward, back straight and knees pointed in the same direction as your feet.

☐ Return to the starting position and repeat.

DUMBBELL INCLINE BENCH PRESS: Pecs, triceps, shoulders

☐ Follow the same instructions as for dumbbell bench press, but lift the backrest of the press bench to 30-45 degrees from flat.

DUMBBELL INCLINE CURL: Biceps

☐ Sit on a press bench with the back angled 30–45 degrees from flat. Hold a dumbbell in each arm, hands hanging down to your sides, palms facing forwards. This is your starting position.

☐ Bend both arms, pulling the dumbbells up towards your head. Don't let them touch and try not to use your back or momentum to carry them upwards. Hold at the top for a moment and slowly lower back down to the starting position.

DUMBBELL REVERSE LUNGES: Quads, hamstrings, glutes

☐ Start in a standing position holding some dumbbells by your sides. Look forward, keeping your chest up, with your feet shoulder-width apart.

☐ Start the movement by taking a large step to the rear. Allow your knee and hip to flex so your body lowers. Descend until your knee almost touches the ground. Aim to keep the movement controlled and focus on proper posture. The knee should stay in line with the foot.

☐ Drive through the heel of the front leg to extend the knees and hips and return to the starting position.

DUMBBELL SHOULDER PRESS: Shoulders

☐ Hold a dumbbell in each hand. Sit on a bench that has an upright back support. Raise the dumbbells to shoulder height one at a time using your lower body to help get them up into position.

☐ Rotate your wrists so that your palms are facing forward. This is your starting position.

☐ Push the dumbbells upward until they touch at the top when your arms are fully extended. Slowly lower the weights back down to the starting position.

☐ Repeat for the recommended number of repetitions.

DUMBBELL STEP-UPS: Quads, hamstrings, glutes

☐ Stand up straight, holding a dumbbell in each hand by your sides, with a bench/step in front of you. Step one foot up on the elevated platform, lift the rest of your body up and place the foot of the other leg on the platform as well.

☐ Step down using the same leg first. Return to the original standing position and repeat, leading with the same foot, until you have done the required number of reps. When you have finished, repeat on the other side, leading with the other foot.

DUMBBELL THRUSTER: Shoulders, quads, hamstrings, glutes

☐ Lift two dumbbells to shoulder height. Keep the weights close to your shoulders. Rotate your wrists so your palms are facing inwards. This is your starting position.

☐ Start a squat by flexing with your hips and knees. Aim on staying upright with a straight back as you descend.

☐ At the bottom of the squat, reverse the movement and drive up by extending your knees and hips. As you do this, press both the dumbbells overhead by extending your arms straight up. You can use the momentum from the squat to drive the weights upward.

☐ Lower the weight back to shoulder height to begin the next repetition.

HAMMER CURLS: Biceps

☐ Start in a standing position with a dumbbell in each hand. Arms should be by your sides with your palms facing inward. Look ahead, with your chest up and your feet shoulder-width apart.

☐ Flex the elbows to curl the weight up to

shoulder-height, keeping your palms facing inwards. Do not rely on momentum or use the shoulders. Finish with the dumbbells just below your ears.

☐ Reverse the motion slowly to return to the starting position.

KETTLEBELL DEADLIFTS: Lower back, hamstrings, glutes, quads

☐ Start in a standing position with a kettlebell held with both hands. Your back should be slightly arched and ensure you maintain this through the movement.

☐ Start the movement by slowly pushing your hips back and letting the weight travel down your legs to your shins. The knees should only bend slightly. Keep the weight on the heels. Maintain the arch in your back throughout the exercise as you lower, keeping the weight tight to your legs. Don't round your shoulders at the bottom of the movement.

☐ When you reach the bottom of the movement, return to the starting position by extending the hips, finishing upright, weight over the hips.

KETTLEBELL GOBLET SQUAT: Quads, hamstrings

☐ Stand holding a kettlebell by its handle using both hands, close to your chest. This is your starting position.

☐ Squat down by flexing your knees and hips until you reach the bottom of the squat

position. Keep your chest and head up and your back straight. Continue all the way down until your thighs are just passed parallel to the ground, keeping the weight on the front of the heel. At the bottom of the movement, reverse the motion, driving the weight upward.

KETTLEBELL SINGLE ARM CLEAN AND PRESS: Full body, shoulders

☐ Start by standing with your legs shoulder-width apart. Place a kettlebell on the floor in front of you. Grip it by its handle with an overhand grip, using one hand, palm back.

☐ 'Clean' or lift the kettlebell by swinging it from your legs, bending at the elbow and pulling it towards the shoulder. Hold it at your shoulder and squat down, keeping the torso upright.

☐ Explosively drive through the heels to reverse the squat to standing. Use the body's momentum to extend your arm at the same time to press the weight overhead. Lower the kettlebell to your shoulder then back to the ground to start the next rep. Keep your back straight or slightly arched back throughout the full movement.

KETTLEBELL SWINGS: Hamstrings, glutes

☐ Grab the kettlebell with both hands. Push your hips back and bend your knees to get into the starting position. Keep your back flat. Swing the kettlebell back between your legs. Reverse the direction quickly and drive through with your hips, taking the kettlebell straight out in front of you. Let the kettlebell swing back between your legs and repeat.

LAT PULL DOWN: Lats, triceps

☐ Sit down on a pull-down machine with a wide bar attached to the top pulley. Grip the bar with the palms facing forward. Bring your torso back so you are leaning back slightly.

☐ Pull the bar down until it reaches your upper chest. Focus on drawing the shoulders and the upper arms down and back while keeping the torso stationary.

☐ Squeeze your shoulder blades together at the bottom of the movement then slowly allow the bar to raise back to the starting position.

LATERAL RAISES: Shoulders, upper back

☐ Stand with a straight torso and dumbbells by your sides at arm's length, with the palms of the hand facing you.

☐ Lift the dumbbells up and out on either side of your body with a slight bend of the elbow, keeping the torso fixed. Continue to go up until your arms are parallel to the floor. Now lower the dumbbells slowly to the starting position.

LEG PRESS: Quads, hamstrings, glutes

☐ Using a leg press machine, sit down and place your legs on the platform directly in front of you at shoulder-width apart. Your knees should be at a 90-degree angle. This is your starting position.

☐ Lower the safety bars holding the weighted platform in place and press the platform all the way up until your legs are fully extended in front of you, pushing mostly through the heels of your feet. Make sure the knees don't lock out at any point.

☐ Ensure to lock the safety pins properly once you are done.

LEG PRESS, SINGLE LEG: Quads, hamstrings, glutes

☐ Follow the same instructions as for the leg press, except instead of placing both legs on the platform, place one on the platform and one flat on the floor. Repeat the exercise for the required number of reps then swap legs.

LUNGE AND SHOULDER PRESS: quads, hamstrings, glutes, deltoids

☐ Start with your feet hip-width apart, shoulders back and chest out. Select two dumbbells and hold them at chest height, shoulder-width apart, with palms facing each other.

□ Take a moderate-length step forwards with one foot, lowering your body to a point in which your rear knee gets close to the floor without touching. Keep your torso in an upright position and keep the front knee in line/over the front foot as you perform the exercise. Then drive through the heel at the bottom of the movement to extend the knee and hip and return to the starting position.

□ Perform the pressing movement from the start position by lifting the arms to press the weight above your head. Pause at the top of the movement before reversing the motion to return to the original position. Then return to the lunge on the alternate leg.

NEGATIVE PULL-UP: Lats, upper and middle back, forewarms, biceps

□ Grab a pull-up bar, palms facing forwards, and lift yourself up so that your chin is above the bar. You can use weighted assistance or a friend to help you up.

□ Slowly lower yourself down to fully hanging over the required time. Try to make this movement gradual. If you cannot maintain the movement over the required time, use a weight assist platform under your feet.

PIVOT BARBELL SHOULDER PRESS: Shoulder, triceps

□ Put a weight on one of the ends of an Olympic barbell. Place the unweighted end of the barbell into a pivot bar mount.

Lift the barbell so the weighted end is at shoulder height. Using one arm, press the barbell up/forwards. Stand in a staggered stance with the opposite leg forward to the arm you are pressing with. Lower the bar slowly back to shoulder height and repeat. When you have completed the required number of reps, switch arms.

□ Note: if your gym does not have a pivot bar mount, do a single dumbbell shoulder press instead.

PIVOT BARBELL SINGLE ARM ROW: Lats, upper, middle back

□ Put a weight on one of the ends of an Olympic barbell. Place the other end of the barbell in a pivot bar mount.

□ Stand with the bar between your legs, facing towards the weighted end. Bend forwards until your torso is as close to parallel with the floor as you can manage comfortably. Keep your knees soft.

□ Grip the bar with one hand just behind the plate(s) and put your other hand on your knee. Pull the bar straight until the plates touch your lower chest, keeping the elbow in throughout.

□ Slowly lower the bar back to the starting position. Repeat for the recommended amount of repetitions and switch arms.

□ Note: if your gym does not have a pivot bar mount, replace this exercise with a dumbbell single arm row instead.

PULL-UPS: Lats, upper and middle back, forearms, biceps

- ☐ Start by grabbing a bar with your palms facing forward in a neutral position, around shoulder-width apart. Extend both arms in front of you while holding onto the bar. Aim to have a slight curvature in your back while sticking your chest out. Lift your feet of the ground, then pull your torso up until the top of the chest reaches the bar. From this position drop down to the original starting position in a controlled motion.

- ☐ If you find it too difficult to completed the required number of reps, feel free to use an assistance platform under your feet.

REAR DELT RAISE: Shoulders, mid back

- ☐ Start seated on the end of a bench with your legs together and the dumbbells behind your calves. Bend from the waist, keeping the back straight. Pick up the dumbbells with your palms facing each other. Lift the dumbbells straight up and out on either side of your body until both of your arms are parallel to the floor. Pause for one second at the top, then slowly lower the dumbbells back to the starting position.

RENEGADE ROW: Triceps, pecs, lats, traps, deltoids, abs

- ☐ Hold a dumbbell in both hands (preferably hexagonal/square dumbbells) and get into the push-up position, supporting your weight on the handles of the dumbbells.

- ☐ Shift your bodyweight to one arm and lift the other directly upwards, keeping your arm in line with your body, until the dumbbell is level with your chest. Hold for a moment, then lower to the ground. Repeat for the required number of reps then swap arms.

SEATED ROW: Back, biceps

- ☐ Sit at a low pulley row machine with a V-bar. Place your feet flat on the floor, knees at 90-degrees. Reach forward to grab the V-bar, then sit upright holding the bar with a straight back and arms straight out in front of you. This is your starting position.

- ☐ Breathe out as you pull the bar towards you, keeping your forearms close to your body. Try not to move your torso. Hold for a moment then straighten your arms back to the starting position.

SINGLE ARM ROWS: Lats, upper and middle back, biceps

- ☐ Place your right knee and palm on a bench, your left foot on the floor and a dumbbell in your left hand, arm hanging down.

- ☐ Bend your left arm, bringing the elbow backwards keeping the arm in line with your body, until your elbow is level with your head. Hold for a second then lower. Repeat for the required number of reps, then swap arms.

SWISS BALL ATOMIC PUSH-UP:
Full body, core, chest

☐ Start by lying on the floor face down, placing your hands shoulder-width apart and holding your upper body up at an arm's length. Place your toes on top of an exercise ball. This will raise your body into an elevated posistion. Then lower yourself until your chest has almost touched the floor. Using your chest muscles, press your upper body back up to the starting position. Keep the back straight with the core engaged.

SWISS BALL HAMSTRING CURLS: Hamstrings

☐ Start by lying on the floor on your back with your feet raised up on top of the Swiss ball. Position the ball so that when your legs are fully extended your ankles are resting on the top of it. From there, raise your hips off the ground, keeping your weight in your shoulders and your feet. With the knees flexed, start pulling the ball as close to you as you can, using the hamstrings. After a short pause at the top, return to the starting position.

SWISS BALL ROLL-OUT: Abs, core

☐ Start in a kneeling position on a mat with your forearms resting on top of the Swiss ball. Roll the ball forward slowly, from your forearms to your elbows as far as you can, keeping your back in a neutral position. Keeping the core engaged, roll the ball back to the starting position.

TRICEP DIPS: Triceps

☐ Using parallel bars, holding your body off the ground with your arms nearly locked above the bars. Now slowly lower yourself downward. Your body should remain upright with your elbows staying close to your body. Lower yourself down until a 90-degree angle is formed with the upper arm and forearm.

☐ Then push your torso back up using your triceps, bringing yourself back to the starting position.

☐ If this is too difficult, use an assistance platform under your feet, or replace with bench dips (see Home-based resistance plan) until you are strong enough.

TRICEP PUSH-DOWN: Triceps

☐ Using a rope attachment on a high pulley, grab the handles with palms facing away. Hold your arms at your sides, with your elbows at 90 degrees, forearms pointing forwards. This is your starting position.

☐ Keeping a straight back, straighten your arms so your hands are just in front of your hips. Hold for a moment before slowly returning to the starting position.

CARDIO: LISS

These activities should be 15–60 minutes in duration, and as the name suggests they should be low intensity in order to target the fat-burning zone of exercise. There are two ways to make sure you're in the fat-burning zone when exercising:

#1 Heart Rate: this is a great tool if you have a heart rate monitor (I recommend using a chest strap rather than wrist sensor, as wrist sensors can be very unreliable). You should be aiming for a heart rate of around 60–65% of your maximum heart rate (MHR). You can calculate your MHR approximately with this calculation: 220 – age in years. To get 60% you multiply this number by 0.6 and to get 65% you multiply by 0.65. If this is too much maths for you (it is for me!) then here is a handy table for a range of ages, rounded to the nearest decimal point:

Age	60%-65%				
20	120-130	33	112-122	47	104-112
21	119-129	34	112-121	48	103-112
22	119-129	35	111-120	49	103-111
23	118-128	36	110-120	50	102-111
24	118-127	37	110-119	51	101-110
25	117-127	38	109-118	52	101-109
26	116-126	39	109-118	53	100-109
27	116-125	40	108-117	54	100-108
28	115-125	41	107-116	55	99-107
29	115-124	42	107-116	56	98-107
30	114-124	43	106-115	57	98-106
31	113-123	44	106-114	58	97-105
32	113-122	45	105-114	59	97-105
		46	104-113	60	96-104

#2 Perceived exertion: if you don't have a heart rate monitor, you can make a good estimate of your exercise zone from the level of effort you feel like you're putting in.

In the fat-burning zone, you should find that you can hold a simple conversation, but it's difficult to make long sentences without getting out of breath. If you get to the point where you can only say one or two words at a time, you're pushing too hard. You should notice your breathing is fairly heavy and that you're sweating.

EXERCISE SELECTION

The movements you can do within this range will vary depending slightly on your fitness levels. If you have high levels of fitness then a steady jog may fit at this level, if you are less fit then a power walk would be more suitable as an example. I typically prefer either a power walk or a gentle cycle: personally these keep me in the right zone.

Here are the options I often use. Feel free to select any movements from this list or any others you might prefer that keep you in the zone:

- ☐ **Cross-trainer**
- ☐ **Cycling**
- ☐ **Power walking**
- ☐ **Air bike**
- ☐ **Rowing**
- ☐ **Swimming**

CARDIO: INTERVAL TRAINING

We covered the benefits of interval training on page 185– here's how you can include them in your plan.

TABATA

Tabata is a short, sharp and simple format that helps boost fitness and adds some extra intensity. These sessions have gained a huge amount of popularity recently.

The format of the session is 20-seconds work and 10-seconds rest for 8 rounds, so 4 minutes overall. This means the 20-seconds need to be done at a very high intensity.

The criterion of this type of training is that the 20 seconds should be at 170% of your VO2 max – that means the maximum volume of oxygen you can utilise during intense, or maximal exercise. VO2 max is difficult to measure so we will rely on how you feel. If you feel OK afterwards you've not done it properly, you should feel exhausted! The first three efforts will feel hard but the last two will feel impossibly hard. The plan is for 8 rounds, but sometimes it may be hard to survive all 8 so I'll let you off with 7.

Due to the intensity of these sessions movement selection is important. Some people do it with sit-ups, skipping, jogging on the spot and bodyweight squats, but these simply do not allow for enough intensity. I recommend one of the following:

- ☐ **Spin bike**
- ☐ **Air bike**
- ☐ **Rowing**
- ☐ **Track running**

While you will struggle to hit the true intensity needed to match the researched study, these exercises will allow for a suitable intensity to provide results.

RUSSIAN STEPS

This session is similarly short and sharp, it challenges your body for varying lengths of intervals and is very effective for boosting intensity and fat burning.

The format of this session is like a ladder or a boomerang – with short intervals and rest building to longer intervals and rest and then back down the other way:

15 seconds work, 15 seconds rest
30 seconds work, 30 seconds rest
45 seconds work, 45 seconds rest
60 seconds work, 60 seconds rest
45 seconds work, 45 seconds rest
30 seconds work, 30 seconds rest
15 seconds work, 15 seconds rest

This works out to 16 minutes of exercise. The work blocks should be at high intensity, while the rests should be low intensity. I recommend the same exercises as for Tabata, to ensure you can push to a high enough intensity.

CIRCUIT TRAINING: AKA DECK OF CARDS

Over the past 7–8 years I would say my deck of cards workout has been one of the most popular parts of the plan. It's a fun twist on traditional circuits. This is how it works:

☐ Take a pack of cards (make sure the jokers are still included),

☐ Choose a routine from the table below.

☐ Shuffle the deck very well and pull a card from the top. The number on the card is the number of reps for the exercise. Picture cards are 10 reps. Aces are 11 reps. The joker is a well-needed 1 minute rest.

☐ Work through all 54 of the cards – although if you are new to fitness, I would suggest working through half the deck initially, with one joker.

So for example, let's say you picked Beginner Routine 1, and drew the following cards: **7♦, K♣, A♥, 2♥, 3♠, 4♠, J♠, ✹Joker**
You would do 7 Dips, 10-seconds of Glute bridge, 11 Squats, 17 Star Jumps, then a 1-minute rest.

BEGINNER	INTERMEDIATE
ROUTINE 1:	**ROUTINE 1:**
♥ Hearts – **Squats**	♥ Hearts – **Squats**
♦ Diamonds – **Dips**	♦ Diamonds – **Push-ups**
♣ Clubs – **Glute bridge (seconds)**	♣ Clubs – **Squat thrusts**
♠ Spades – **Star jumps**	♠ Spades – **Shuttle runs (10m)**
✹ Joker – 1-min rest	✹ Joker – 1-min rest
ROUTINE 2:	**ROUTINE 2:**
♥ Hearts – **Squats**	♥ Hearts – **Lunges (each leg)**
♦ Diamonds – **Walking plank**	♦ Diamonds – **Push-ups**
♣ Clubs – **Mountain climbers (seconds)**	♣ Clubs – **Burpees**
♠ Spades – **Star jumps**	♠ Spades – **Step-ups (each leg)**
✹ Joker – 1-min rest	✹ Joker – 1-min rest

LET'S GET FITTER, FASTER!

We've made it! I doubt you've ever been more ready, more committed or more motivated to make a very real tangible difference to your health and fitness than you are now. I know I've given you a lot of information to get you here, but I genuinely believe that it's important.

I cannot wait to see where you take everything you've learned and how you progress, not just over the next 8 weeks, but over the next 8 years and beyond.

This book was always designed to give you more than just some nice recipes and a couple of exercises. It was never about short-term fixes. I wanted to prime you for success for the rest of your life. Now, you've got your personalised plan, you're ready to go. You're armed with everything you need to succeed. Put simply:

THIS PLAN + YOUR DEDICATION × OUR COMMITMENT = SUCCESS

A few points to remember before I let you loose to smash your goals:

- Fitness results come from consistency, not all-out effort over a short period of time. The best results are built through changes in lifestyle: making healthy eating and exercise part of your everyday routine.
- To be consistent, you need to follow both your exercise and plan week in, week out. Don't let small problems become big ones. Stay focused and keep on track.
- You have everything you need in this plan to achieve great results. It will work if you follow it consistently and with focus.

As a parting gift to help you succeed, I want you to complete the form on the next page. It will help you if you reread it at times when you're feeling less motivated than you are now.

What will be your biggest challenge following the food plan in this book?

....

....

How will you overcome it?

....

....

What will be your biggest challenge following the exercise plan in this book?

....

....

How will you overcome it?

....

....

If I achieve 7 consecutive days following the food plan perfectly, I will reward myself with (non-food related)

....

If I achieve 14 consecutive days following the exercise plan perfectly I will reward myself with (non-food related)

....

I know now what you will know in eight weeks time. You are destined for greatness and you are going to achieve more in the next eight weeks than you can possibly imagine. I wish I could prove it to you right now, but you're going to prove it to me.

Take a photo of what you look like now and then another in 8 weeks. Send them both to me at fitterfaster@davidkingsbury.co.uk. Look at them side by side and then tell me you don't look better and feel better than you ever have before.

MEETING YOUR EXPECTATIONS

I believe in this plan. I believe in you and I hope that, by now, you are starting to believe in yourself. This plan will work for you if you embrace it and all its ideals.

I'm writing this chapter for those of you for whom this plan may not be going perfectly. It's hidden way at the back, like a special little club where its location is only known by a select few. The first rule of this Chapter is that we don't talk about this Chapter . . . except we do. We have to. If you've wandered into this chapter by accident and you're doing great, then move along. There's nothing to see here.

Over the course of this plan, there will be times when you might doubt the changes your body is undergoing. You might not be seeing the results you were expecting when you look in the mirror. Before you give up, have a read of the below. As human beings our bodies adhere to the Energy Balance Equation: each and every one of us is governed by the laws of physics. If you haven't lost weight, then you have not been in a calorie deficit. It is as simple as that. Let's look at some of the reasons you might not be hitting your calorie deficit.

#1 YOU'RE NOT BEING HONEST WITH YOURSELF ON HOW MANY CALORIES YOU ARE CONSUMING This is the most common
cause for slow or non-existent progress. While you're on the plan, keeping on track of what you are eating, and what you need to eat, is crucial. It is so easy for additional, unexpected calories to creep up and, before you know it, you have exceeded your calorie limit for the day. Think about that cheeky little biscuit with your cuppa, the cakes at work that arrive for someone's birthday or those free nibbles in the supermarket. A lot of the time those extra calories can be found in perfectly healthy food, but even healthy foods are not calorie free! These are a few popular foods that seem healthy, but are actually calorie-dense, that might be tipping you into the positive energy balance without you realising it. Things like nuts, nut butter, coconut oil, avocados, oils, dried food and dried chocolate.

As well as healthy foods being a calorie boost, unhealthy foods also may be responsible. If there is any junk food or processed food slipping into your days, then they are more than likely responsible for the lack of progress. If you thought one cheeseburger wouldn't matter, it's time to think again!

#2 LIQUID CALORIES AREN'T BEING COUNTED Liquid calories is one reason people are gaining body fat in the first place. It's best to avoid them where you can. It's not just alcohol, though, all those caffè lattes, fruit juices or even 'flavoured' water, can all add some serious calories to your day. A large latte, for example, will be pushing on for 200 calories. If you have a couple of these every day, they will easily take you out of your fat loss zone and right up into maintenance, or even weight gain.

#3 YOU'VE MISCALCULATED YOUR CALORIES This is something that is very simple to do. When you calculated your own calories targets in Part 1, it could be as simple as a small mathematical miscalculation. I would recommend going back and recalculating your number. You may well find that, if you have got your weight wrong or miscalculated your activity level, a simple redo will get you back on track.

#4 YOU AREN'T MEASURING YOUR WEIGHT OVER SEVERAL DAYS AND TAKING AN AVERAGE Your bodyweight fluctuates daily by several kilos for many reasons. To get an accurate idea of how much you really weigh, you need to make sure you measure yourself over at least 3 days and take an average.

#5 YOUR BODY HAS BECOME LESS EFFICIENT If you have been on the plan for 4 weeks or so and you've been following it closely without straying from the menu and you still haven't lost weight or are not losing as much weight as you would like to, then this section is for you. Losing weight and gaining weight are accompanied by biological changes that you won't necessarily be aware of, some of which may mean that you might be expending slightly less energy than would be based on predicted calories. If you have been through a diet-then-weight-gain process several times in the past, your base level calories may have dropped slightly. But don't worry, fat loss is still possible. Use the below formula for your next calorie calculation. If after a couple of weeks on this plan weight still isn't budging then I suggest you up your exercise to create more of a calorie deficit.

FAT-LOSS CALORIES, MALE

Level 1 (hours of exercise per week: 1–3)

Your weight in kg × 11.5 + 585 = Fat-loss calories

Level 2 (hours of exercise per week: 3–5)

Your weight in kg × 14.1 + 725 = Fat-loss calories

Level 3 (hours of exercise per week: 5+)

Your weight in kg × 16.7 + 865 = Fat-loss calories

FAT-LOSS CALORIES, FEMALE

Level 1 (hours of exercise per week: 1–3)

Your weight in kg × 7.7 + 620 = Fat-loss calories

Level 2 (hours of exercise per week: 3–5)

Your weight in kg × 10.0 + 800 = Fat-loss calories

Level 3 (hours of exercise per week: 5+)

Your weight in kg × 12.3 + 985 = Fat-loss calories

#6 YOU'VE LOST WEIGHT SO YOUR CALORIE REQUIREMENT HAS CHANGED If you've lost weight since starting this plan, but haven't recalculated your calories, your results will plateau. As you lose weight, you need to adjust your menu accordingly. Go back to the section on calculating calories and put in your new weight.

WHAT IF I AM LOSING WEIGHT TOO QUICKLY?

Losing weight too quickly can be an issue for quite a lot of people. If you are naturally very active or have a seemingly 'fast metabolism' then this could be you. If you are losing more weight than you want to then you can use the below calculation to increase your calories slightly to slow down weight loss. If after using this formula for a couple of weeks you still find yourself losing too much weight then I suggest you manually increase your calorie by selecting a food plan that is another 100–200 higher than what the above calculation estimates you need. If after using this formula for a couple of weeks you still find yourself losing too much weight then I suggest you manually increase your calorie by selecting a food plan that is another 100–200 higher than what the above calculation estimates you need.

FAT-LOSS CALORIES, MALE

Level 1 (hours of exercise per week: 1–3)
Your weight in kg × 12.6 + 645 = Fat-loss calories

Level 2 (hours of exercise per week: 3–5)
Your weight in kg × 15.5 + 800 = Fat-loss calories

Level 3 (hours of exercise per week: 5+)
Your weight in kg × 19.2 + 985 = Fat-loss calories

FAT-LOSS CALORIES, FEMALE

Level 1 (hours of exercise per week: 1–3)
Your weight in kg × 8.5 + 685 = Fat-loss calories

Level 2 (hours of exercise per week: 3–5)
Your weight in kg × 11.1 + 880 = Fat-loss calories

Level 3 (hours of exercise per week: 5+)
Your weight in kg × 13.5 + 1085 = Fat-loss calories

KEY WORDS AND TERMS

Anabolic

In relationship to fitness, anabolic means the process of building muscle from proteins and nutrients.

Androgens

Androgens are hormones, often referred to as 'male hormones' but are present in both men and women, although in different amounts. The main androgens are testosterone and androstenedione (although there are more).

Calorie

A calorie is a term many of us know or have heard of, but have not always understood what it is. A calorie is a unit of energy in food or drink. It is sometimes referred to as a kilocalorie (or kcal). They are one and the same.

Carbohydrates

Carbohydrates (or carbs) are sugars that break down in the body to create glucose. This glucose is then moved around the body to create fuel for the muscles, brain and other essential biological functions. There are two types of carbs: simple and complex. As the name suggests, simple carbohydrates refer to those sugars with a simple molecular structure that may have only one or two parts. Complex carbs have three or more parts and have a much more complex molecular structure. Because there are more 'parts' the body takes longer to break them down to produce glucose.

Catabolic

While anabolic refers to the process of building muscle, catabolic is the opposite of that. Catabolic refers to breaking down muscle, which can happen, for example, through overtraining.

Cholesterol

Cholesterol, also known as lipid, is a fatty substance vital to the body's normal function. While it can be found in food, it is also mainly made by the liver. It is carried around the body in the blood by proteins. Once combined with protein, it is known as lipoprotein and there are two types; high- (HDL) and low-density lipoprotein (LDL). HDL is commonly referred to as 'good cholesterol' as it is carried away from the cells and back to the liver to be broken down and passed as waste. LDL carries cholesterol to the cells that need it, but if there is more than needed, it builds up on the walls of your arteries. For this reason, it's often called 'bad cholesterol'.

Cortisol

Cortisol, or the 'stress hormone', is the hormone that is released into the bloodstream when we feel stressed. Both the adrenal and pituitary glands, together with the hypothalamus, secrete cortisol when we are under pressure (or stressed), which increased the flow of glucose to your bloodstream and to your tissue. This automatic process can impact on all your bodily functions, including blood sugar levels, blood pressure and fat, protein and carbohydrate metabolism. Excess cortisol over a long period of time can damage the way our bodies utilise glucose.

Energy Balance Equation

The balance in your body between energy in and energy out, which governs whether you lose or gain weight.

Energy In is the sum of the calories from the food and drink you consume.

Energy Out is thesum of your Metabolic Rate, Non-Exercise Activity Thermogenesis (NEAT), Exercise Activity Thermogenesis (EAT) and the Thermic Effect of Food (TEF).

> If Energy In > Energy Out, you will gain weight
>
> If Energy In < Energy Out, you will lose weight

EPOC

EPOC stands for Excess Post-exercise Oxygen Consumption and refers to the amount of oxygen that the body consumes following exercise in excess to the level BEFORE exercising. Just as our body uses more oxygen after exercise than before, it also expends more calories during the post-workout recovery than it did before. The length of time that EPOC is in effect varies depending on the exercise that has been completed, but can help fat loss for hours after your workout has finished.

Glycogen

Glycogen is produced by the liver and is stored either in the liver or the muscle cells. It's the main way that the body stores glucose. Most of the carbs we eat ultimately become glucose.

Hypothalamus

The hypothalamus is a part of the brain, about the size of a pea, that helps to keep the body in a stable condition. It also helps to control many bodily functions including the release of hormones from the pituitary gland, like changes in cortisol levels and body temperature. It can respond to signals from other areas of the body like hunger and feeling full, but also stress levels and blood pressure.

Insulin

Insulin is a hormone made by the pancreas and is released into the bloodstream by beta-cells. Its main role is to control how the body uses carbs and fats found in the food you eat.

Intermittent Fasting

This can be a valuable tool for taking your results that one step further. It works by setting yourself a set eating window each day, within which you consume all your meals and calories, then you fast during the remaining hours of the day. It might sound hard, but it isn't really that bad, and it can really help improve your fat loss potential. So, while it's not essential on this plan and may not be necessary for everyone, it can provide a useful tool for many. See page 39 for more details.

Interval Training

Interval training is a form of cardiovascular training that features periods of varying intensity. Interval training is an effective tool for burning calories, due to the intensity and extra demand for energy. By taking part in interval training, your body and metabolism functions at a higher rate not only while you're doing them, but also for hours afterwards. It's working on your body, even when you're not. The EPOC effect (afterburn from exercise) might not be huge, but it all adds up. The bursts of increased intensity increase calorie expenditure and therefore the total number of calories burned increases.

Low Intensity Steady State Cardio (LISS)

LISS exercises cover any form of low intensity exercise done over a prolonged period of time which increases your heart rate. This could be aerobic exercises such as walking, cycling and swimming if they are performed at a low intensity. Your target heart rate zone for LISS should be between 55% and 70% of maximum heart rate, ideally 60–65%.

Macronutrient (aka Macros)

Macros are what make up the calorie content of our food. Macronutrients come in three categories; carbohydrates, protein and fat. Each of these three combine to make the calorie content of food; 1 gram of carbohydrates is 4 calories, 1 gram of fat is 9 and a gram of protein is 4 calories. Your menu is customised to work synergistically with your body type and your own activity levels. We can accelerate fat loss by either reducing carbohydrates or cycling them within your menu. This will also improve your long-term hormone function.

Metabolism / Metabolic Rate

Simply put, metabolism is the name of the process by which your body converts the food and drink you eat, combining it with oxygen, into energy. Your body needs energy for even the most basic functions such as breathing, repairing damaged cells and circulating blood around the body, and the number of calories your body uses to carry out these functions is known as your basal metabolic rate. There are other factors that impact on this rate, such as gender, age, body size and composition.

Non-Exercise Activity Thermogenesis (NEAT)

The calories your body burns due to activity, but not deliberate exercise. This includes wandering around, shopping and fidgeting.

Resistance Training

Resistance training is an exercise where you move your body against resistance, i.e. any force that makes the movement harder to perform. Resistance can be provided simply by performing movements against gravity or by adding weight. Resistance can also be added using gym machines, or by using equipment such as weighted bars, bands, or kettlebells.

RECIPE INDEX

Ham, egg and avocado with honey mustard 177

Ham, potato, onion and spinach frittata 65

Honey yogurt with flaked almonds 167

Huevos rancheros 60

Kale and pork with sautéed apple 123

Matcha apple green shake 168

Mexican spice bowl 78

Mixed bean salad with yogurt 151

Mozzarella, ham and tomatoes with Med. drizzle 178

New York-style open pastrami and turkey sandwich 94

Paprika prawn cocktail pot 167

Prawn Thai green curry 112

Protein bircher bowls 133

Protein carrot cake 146

Raspberry almond pancakes 58

Raspberry chia pudding 50

Salmon and roast veg 111

Salmon eggs royale with yogurt hollandaise 71

Salmon pasta salad with lemon and capers 98

Scrambled egg, turkey bacon, spinach and rye 68

Seitan 'meatballs' with veg and tomato sauce 86

Simple cinnamon peanut protein shake 176

Smoked salmon, cream cheese and cucumber on rice cakes 156

Steak and eggs, with sweet potato hash and sautéed spinach 67

Steak and roast vegetables 103

Sushi bowl 83

Sweet potato chips with tuna dip 152

Tempeh pad Thai with shirataki noodles 100

Toast with spinach and chicken in herb mayo 145

Tuna and asparagus with kidney beans 128

Tuna and bean stir-fry 120

Tuna bean salad 77

Tuna-stuffed courgette 104

Tuna-stuffed peppers 90

Turkey and egg ramen 127

Turkey, bacon, spinach and sweet potato quiche 74

Turkey, bacon, spinach and sweet potato quiche 74

Yogurt and whey 164

GENERAL INDEX

ACKNOWLEDGEMENTS

Firstly, I'd like to say thank you to everyone who has trusted me to be their personal trainer over the years and that now includes you. Thank you for inspiring me every day.

I'd also like to thank a few people who have helped me bring this book to life.

I have an incredible team around me. This book has been a labour of love, but it has also been a team effort, so I'd like to say thanks to my wife, Kirsty, my daughter, Isla and my son, Charlie, for all their support and patience. Also, I want to thank my team, in particular Mark, Chris, Gary and Jonnie. I wouldn't be able to do what I do without your help.

I would also like to thank the incredible team at Orion: Amanda Harris, Emily Barrett, Helen Ewing, Clare Sivell, Alice Commins and Katie Horrocks. As well as the shoot team, whose amazing talent brought the food to life in these pages: Sam Folan, Lou Kenney, Lauren Miller and Charlotte Gaskell.

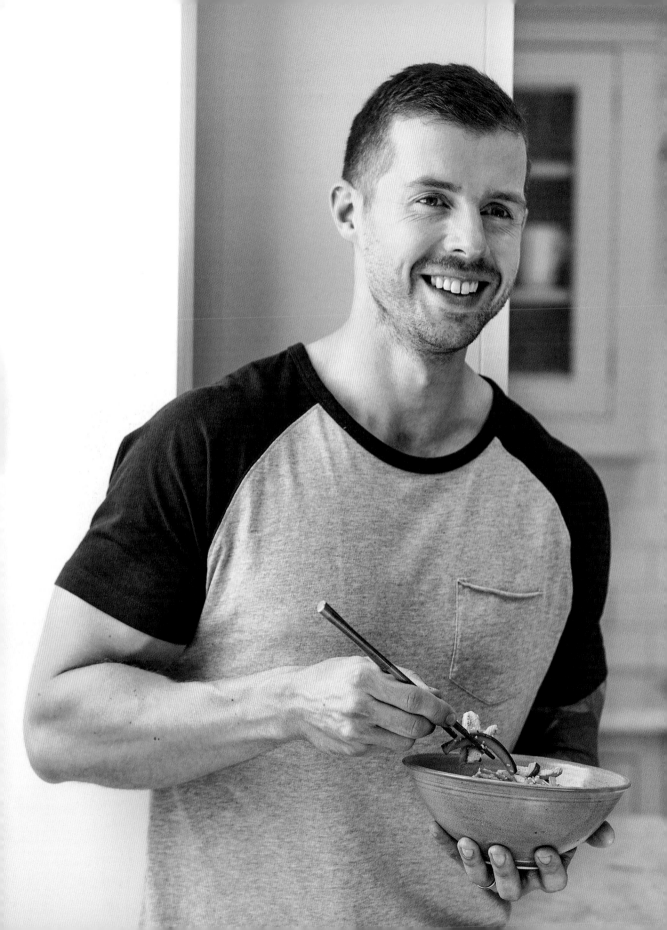

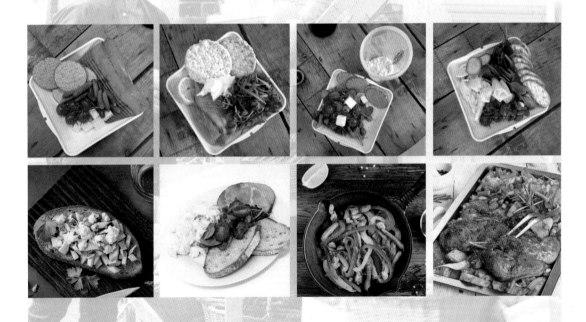

First published in Great Britain in 2018
by Seven Dials,
An imprint of the Orion Publishing Group Ltd
Carmelite House
50 Victoria Embankment
London EC4Y 0DZ
An Hachette UK Company

1 3 5 7 9 10 8 6 4 2

A CIP catalogue record for this book
is available from the British Library.

ISBN: 9781409174776

Photography: Sam Folan
Food stylist: Lou Kenney
Prop stylist: Lauren Miller
Design: Clare Sivell and Rich Carr
Grooming: Charlotte Gaskell
Printed in Italy

Every effort has been made to ensure that the information in this book is accurate and up-to-date at the
time of publication, however information regarding nutrition and training is constantly evolving and the
application of it to particular circumstances depends on many factors. The information in this book may not
be applicable in each individual case so it is advised that professional medical advice is obtained for specific
health matters. Neither the publisher nor author accepts any legal responsibility for any personal injury
or other damage or loss arising from the use of the information in this book. You should always consult a
health practitioner first before changing your diet or exercise regime.

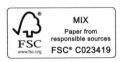

www.orionbooks.co.uk

For more delicious recipes plus exclusive competitions and sneak previews
from Orion's cookery writers visit kitchentales.co.uk

Follow us

@kitchentalesuk

@kitchentalesuk

@kitchentalesuk

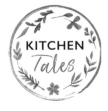